SECOND EDITION

Davis's
Basic Math Review
For Nursing and
Health Professions

with Step-by-Step Solutions

D0217170

SECOND EDITION

Davis's
Basic Math Review
For Nursing and
Health Professions
with *Step-by-Step Solutions*

Vicki Raines, BS, PTCB
Learning Specialist, Educational Assistance Center
Math Instructor, Adult Education
Temple College
Temple, Texas

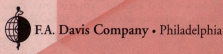

F.A. Davis Company • Philadelphia

F. A. Davis Company
1915 Arch Street
Philadelphia, PA 19103
www.fadavis.com

Copyright © 2017 by F. A. Davis Company

Copyright © 2010, 2017. All rights reserved. This book is protected by copyright. No part of it may be reproduced, stored in a retrieval system, or transmitted in any form or by any means, electronic, mechanical, photocopying, recording, or otherwise, without written permission from the publisher.

Printed in the United States of America
Last digit indicates print number: 10 9 8 7 6 5 4 3 2 1

Senior Acquisitions Editor: Megan Klim
Senior Content Project Manager: Elizabeth Hart
Digital Project Manager: Sandra Glennie
Design and Illustration Manager: Carolyn O'Brien

As new scientific information becomes available through basic and clinical research, recommended treatments and drug therapies undergo changes. The author(s) and publisher have done everything possible to make this book accurate, up to date, and in accord with accepted standards at the time of publication. The author(s), editors, and publisher are not responsible for errors or omissions or for consequences from application of the book, and make no warranty, expressed or implied, in regard to the contents of the book. Any practice described in this book should be applied by the reader in accordance with professional standards of care used in regard to the unique circumstances that may apply in each situation. The reader is advised always to check product information (package inserts) for changes and new information regarding dose and contraindications before administering any drug. Caution is especially urged when using new or infrequently ordered drugs.

Library of Congress Cataloging-in-Publication Data

Names: Raines, Vicki, author.
Title: Davis's basic math review for nurses : with step-by-step solutions /
    Vicki Raines.
Other titles: Basic math review for nurses
Description: 2nd edition. | Philadelphia : F.A. Davis Company, [2017] |
    Includes index.
Identifiers: LCCN 2016044725 | ISBN 9780803656598
Subjects: | MESH: Mathematics | Nurses' Instruction | Problems and Exercises
Classification: LCC RT68 | NLM QA 107.2 | DDC 610.73076—dc23 LC record available at
https://lccn.loc.gov/2016044725

Authorization to photocopy items for internal or personal use, or the internal or personal use of specific clients, is granted by F. A. Davis Company for users registered with the Copyright Clearance Center (CCC) Transactional Reporting Service, provided that the fee of $.25 per copy is paid directly to CCC, 222 Rosewood Drive, Danvers, MA 01923. For those organizations that have been granted a photocopy license by CCC, a separate system of payment has been arranged. The fee code for users of the Transactional Reporting Service is: 8036-2056-8/09 0 + $.25.

Dedication

Special thanks to Tim, Anne, Samantha, Ed, Charles, Tom, Carol, and Julie

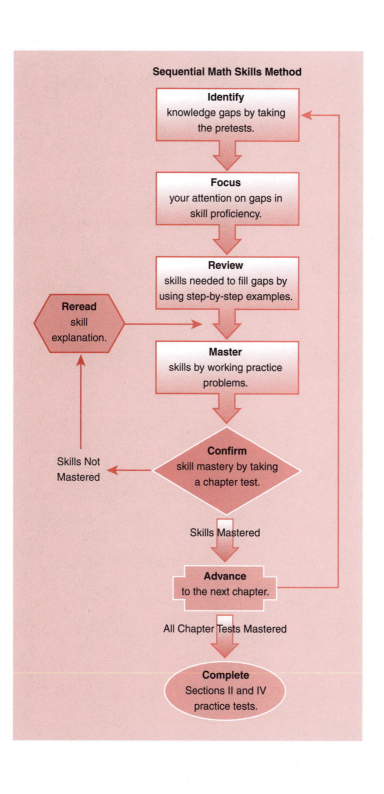

About This Book

Davis's Basic Math Review for Nursing and Health Professions with Step-by-Step Solutions explains the math needed for basic calculations and provides practice problems to help individuals wishing to enter a nursing or health profession field strengthen their math skills. For prospective students, the book provides an excellent review for the math section of any nursing or health profession entrance test.

Davis's Basic Math Review for Nursing and Health Professions with Step-by-Step Solutions presents basic skills in a logical mathematical order so users can easily progress to more advanced skills. For best results, users should work the practice problems and tests in this book without using a calculator because calculators are ***not*** allowed on many of the entrance tests. The more practice problems worked, the faster and more accurate computations become.

Because health care providers often encounter a range of topics requiring math computations—household measures, metric measures, and temperature conversions also are included in this book.

Features of *Davis's Basic Math Review for Nursing and Health Professions with Step-by-Step Solutions*:

- A **pretest** in each chapter helps you determine where to focus your review. Within each pretest is a section number telling you where to find an explanation for that particular skill plus practice problems.
- **Key Terms** are presented in color and are explained in an easy-to-read manner.
- **Math-skill explanations** with example problems are worked step by step to help you understand the skills required.
- **Practice problems** help you master each math skill.
- End of **chapter tests** help you check your progress as you work through the book.
- **Comprehensive practice tests** also help you check for mastery of basic math skills and health care specific applications.

- **Step-by-step solutions** for all pretests, practice problems, chapter tests, and cumulative practice tests help you identify your mistakes and see how to correct your work.
- **Test-Taking Tips** will help you learn how to make the most of your math knowledge and reduce your test-taking anxiety.

For best results with *Davis's Basic Math Review for Nursing and Health Professions with Step-by-Step Solutions,* complete the entire review regardless of your math-skill level. By doing so, you can enhance speed and accuracy in your math computations.

Tips for Taking a Math Test

These tips are divided into three parts: studying for a math test, taking a math test on paper, and taking a standardized math test on a computer. For best test-taking success, follow all suggestions carefully.

Studying for a Math Test

1. Solve all the practice problems, and check your answers for accuracy.
2. Write down and memorize any skill rules the test covers.
3. Review the problems to be covered on the test. Rework several of each type of problem.
4. Review the instructions for the problems. Be sure you understand the wording of the instructions.
5. Complete additional problems or a practice test.
6. Put down your pencil, and work through the review in your mind. Look at each problem, and be sure you know the first step in solving that type of problem. Usually, if you know the first step, you can complete the problem.

Taking a Math Test on Paper

1. As soon as you receive the test, jot down the rules you have memorized.
2. Glance at the problems on the test. A quick scan will tell you which problems may require the most time.
3. Go back to the first problem and start working.
4. If you are unable to solve a problem, write the problem's number at the top of the page and move on. Something later in the test may trigger a solution for the troublesome problem.
5. Continue working problems and writing the number of each troublesome problem at the top of the page.
6. After attempting all of the problems once, go back, and start working the problem(s) listed at the top of each page. If you see your mistake immediately, fix it, and finish solving the problem. But do

not spend time trying to find a mistake. Instead, rewrite the problem on another piece of paper, and start over.

7. Repeat Step 6 until time is up or until you have completed the test.

Preparing for a Standardized Math Test

Ask Questions: *Before taking any standardized test, determine the answers to these questions.*

- Do blank answers count against your score? If so, then making an educated guess is better than leaving any answers blank.
- How many problems are on the test and what is the time limit? By knowing the number of problems and the time limit, you can determine how quickly you will need to work each problem.
- Are you allowed to go back and rework problems if you are taking the test on a computer?
- Are you allowed to use a calculator?

Minimize Distraction, Maximize Concentration: Some testing environments are noisy, and earplugs may be beneficial. If you decide to use earplugs—buy, wear, and get used to them long before the test day.

Taking a Standardized Math Test on a Computer

1. After sitting down at the testing computer, arrange your paper and workspace so that you can work comfortably. Place the mouse in a comfortable, useable position.
2. Ask the test proctor any questions that you have about the computer.
3. Read all of the test instructions carefully.
4. Before beginning the test, write **TIME** and **GO BACK (if the test allows you to go back and rework problems)** on your scratch paper.
5. Write your starting time under **TIME** so you can estimate your working rate and stay aware of the remaining time. Some test screens do not provide time remaining information.
6. Write the problems down neatly and quickly. Solve quickly. If your answer is not a choice, glance at the monitor to be sure you copied the problem correctly. Quickly scan your work for an error. If it is better to make an educated guess on the test, then make one. You

might run out of time and not get the opportunity to go back and rework the problem. Write the problem number under **GO BACK.**

7. If you finish working all the problems before the time is up, stop before submitting your answers. This is the time to rework the problems on your **GO-BACK** list.

8. To use your time most efficiently, go back to the highest number (the problem you most recently worked) on your **GO-BACK** list. Then work back to the lowest number if time allows.

Contents

SECOND EDITION

Davis's
Basic Math Review
For Nursing and
Health Professions

with *Step-by-Step Solutions*

Basic Math Skills

part I

1.0   **Pretest for Whole Numbers**

Solve the following problems. After taking the test, see "Step-by-Step Solutions" for the answers (page 219). Then, see "1.1 Adding Whole Numbers," "1.2 Subtracting Whole Numbers," "1.3 Multiplying Whole Numbers," and "1.4 Dividing Whole Numbers," for skill explanations.

Section 1.1

1. $\begin{array}{r} 5{,}057 \\ +\ 8{,}876 \end{array}$

2. $\begin{array}{r} 12{,}672 \\ +\ 9{,}458 \end{array}$

Section 1.2

3. $\begin{array}{r} 4{,}632 \\ -\ 743 \end{array}$

4. $\begin{array}{r} 71{,}043 \\ -\ 68{,}736 \end{array}$

Section 1.3

5. $\begin{array}{r} 578 \\ \times\ 9 \end{array}$

6. $\begin{array}{r} 625 \\ \times\ 79 \end{array}$

7. $\begin{array}{r} 645 \\ \times\ 708 \end{array}$

Section 1.4

Write your answer with a remainder if needed.

8. $17\overline{)759}$

9. $15\overline{)8{,}080}$

10. $236\overline{)10{,}400}$

1

Adding Whole Numbers
In this section, we will review:
- addition terminology
- an easy format for problem-solving
- carrying numbers

Addition Terminology

In addition, the numbers to be added are called **addends.** The answer is called the **sum**.

$$\begin{array}{r} \text{addend} \\ + \text{addend} \\ \hline \text{sum} \end{array}$$

Before adding **whole numbers**, write the problem vertically (up and down), lining up the numbers in the far right column. The columns must line up for the answer to be correct.

437 + 42 should be written as $\begin{array}{r} \mathbf{437} \\ \mathbf{+\ 42} \\ \hline \end{array}$ before beginning to add.

Always start adding with the far right column (the ones' column), and then move left to the next column (the tens' column). Continue until you have added all columns.

Carrying Numbers

In math, we use a base 10-place value system. Therefore, if you have a sum of 10 or greater in any column, you must **carry** a number to the top of the next column to the left. Then, you add the carried number to the numbers in that column. The following examples show you how to carry.

Example 1: 54 + 38

STEP 1. Add 4 + 8. The sum is 12. Write 2 below the 8. Carry the 1. (Write 1 above the 5.)

STEP 2. Add 1 + 5 + 3. The sum is 9. Write 9 to the left of the 2.

The answer is 92.

$$\begin{array}{r} 1 \\ 54 \\ +\ 38 \\ \hline 92 \end{array}$$

Example 2: 476 + 367 + 458

STEP 1. Add 6 + 7 + 8. The sum is 21. Write 1 below
the 8. Carry the 2. (Write 2 above the 7.)
STEP 2. Add 2 + 7 + 6 + 5. The sum is 20. Write 0
below the 5. Carry the 2. (Write 2 above the 4.)
STEP 3. Add 2 + 4 + 3 + 4. The sum is 13. Write 13
to the left of the 0.

The answer is 1,301.

$$\begin{array}{r} ^{2\,2} \\ 476 \\ 367 \\ +\ 458 \\ \hline 1{,}301 \end{array}$$

1.1 Practice Adding Whole Numbers

Solve the following problems. See "Step-by-Step Solutions" (pages 219 to 220) for the answers.

1. 408 + 241	**2.** 523 + 271	**3.** 405 + 561	**4.** 216 + 423

5. 640 + 118	**6.** 7,244 + 2,786	**7.** 8,563 + 4,567	**8.** 5,042 + 1,966

9. 5,787 + 2,344	**10.** 3,329 + 4,783	**11.** 4,815 + 6,396	**12.** 7,586 + 1,645

13. 4,116 + 3,168	**14.** 7,121 + 2,850	**15.** 2,351 + 7,499	**16.** 4,386 3,798 + 1,745

17. 7,038 1,056 + 2,784	**18.** 6,748 5,902 + 4,352	**19.** 8,764 9,989 + 6,478	**20.** 2,697 7,507 + 4,572

Subtracting Whole Numbers
In this section, we will review:
- subtraction terminology
- an easy format for problem-solving
- borrowing numbers

Subtraction Terminology

In subtraction, the larger number is called the **minuend**, the smaller number (or the number being subtracted) is called the **subtrahend**, and the answer is called the **difference**.

$$\begin{array}{r} \text{minuend} \\ - \text{ subtrahend} \\ \hline \text{difference} \end{array}$$

An Easy Format for Problem-Solving

Subtraction is the inverse (opposite) of addition because you take away numbers, and your answer is always smaller than the original number. If you know your addition facts, then you know your subtraction facts.

The first step in a subtraction problem is to write the numbers vertically (up and down) with the larger number at the top. Line up the numbers on the far right as you do when adding. As in addition, always start working subtraction problems in the far right column. Easy subtraction involves using basic subtraction facts.

Example 1:   37 – 25
STEP 1. Subtract 5 from 7. Write 2 below the 5.
STEP 2. Subtract 2 from 3. Write 1 to the left of the 2.
The answer is 12.

$$\begin{array}{r} 37 \\ - 25 \\ \hline 12 \end{array}$$

Borrowing Numbers

In some subtraction problems, the bottom number in a column may be greater than the top number. When this happens, you must **borrow** from a column to the left to make the top number larger. Borrowing several times in one subtraction problem may be necessary as shown in Example 3.

Example 2: 546 – 18

STEP 1. Observe that you cannot subtract 8 from 6. Therefore, you must borrow a 1 from the column to the left of the 6. Cross out the 4 and write a 3 above it. Write 1 in front of the 6 to form 16. Reason: When you borrow a 1 from the 4 in the column to the left of the 6, you actually borrow a 10 (from the tens' column).

STEP 2. Subtract 8 from 16. Write 8 below the 8. Subtract the next column to the left: 3 – 1 = 2. Write 2 below the 1.

STEP 3. Bring down the 5; no number is below it to subtract.

The answer is 528.

$$\begin{array}{r} \overset{3\ 16}{5\cancel{4}6} \\ -\ 18 \\ \hline 528 \end{array}$$

Borrowing from Zero

When a subtraction problem has a zero in the top number, you must borrow unless a zero is directly under it. Keep borrowing until you can subtract. See Example 3.

Example 3: 406 – 159

STEP 1. Determine if you can subtract the number in the far right column. Because you cannot subtract 9 from 6, look one column to the left. The digit to the left of 6 is 0. You cannot borrow from 0. Look to the next number to the left, the 4.

STEP 2. Borrow 1 from the 4. Cross out the 4, and write a 3 above it. Write 1 in front of the 0 (or write 10 above the 0 as shown). Now, the 0 becomes 10.

STEP 3. Look at the far right column again. You still cannot subtract 9 from 6. However, now you can borrow 1 from 10. Cross out the 10 and write a 9 above it. Write a 1 in front of the 6 (or write 16 above the 6 as shown). Now the 6 becomes 16 and you can subtract 9 from 16.

STEP 4. Subtract 9 from 16. Write 7 below the 9. Subtract the next column to the left: 9 – 5 = 4. Write 4 below the 5. Subtract the next column to the left: 3 – 1 = 2. Write 2 below the 1.

The answer is 247.

You will need to borrow twice in this problem.

The first time you borrow:

$$\begin{array}{r} \overset{3\ \cancel{10}}{\cancel{4}06} \\ -\ 159 \end{array}$$

The second time you borrow:

$$\begin{array}{r} \overset{9\ 16}{\underset{}{}} \\ \overset{3\ \cancel{10}}{\cancel{4}\cancel{0}6} \\ -159 \\ \hline 247 \end{array}$$

Solve the following problems. See "Step-by-Step Solutions" (pages 220 to 221) for the answers.

1. 7,642 − 4,210	**2.** 8,235 − 3,123	**3.** 174 − 48	**4.** 347 − 129
5. 692 − 217	**6.** 7,843 − 6,274	**7.** 4,376 − 2,808	**8.** 3,275 − 1,744
9. 3,456 − 2,738	**10.** 3,010 − 2,563	**11.** 7,133 − 2,924	**12.** 5,301 − 3,466
13. 2,007 − 347	**14.** 6,231 − 430	**15.** 5,005 − 4,835	**16.** 9,112 − 2,569
17. 6,002 − 3,574	**18.** 8,303 − 1,227	**19.** 9,041 − 2,961	**20.** 4,000 − 2,564

1.3   **Multiplying Whole Numbers**
In this section, we will review:
- multiplication terminology
- an easy format for problem solving
- partial products
- multiplying by zero

Multiplication Terminology

In multiplication, a **multiplicand** and a **multiplier** are multiplied to find a **product** (the answer). Sometimes, the multiplicand and multiplier are both called **factors**. You will see the latter term used in nursing-specific applications.

$$\begin{array}{r} \text{multiplicand} \\ \times\ \text{multiplier} \\ \hline \text{product} \end{array}$$

The first step in solving a multiplication problem is to write the problem vertically (up and down) as shown, placing the longer number above the shorter number. Line up the numbers in the right-hand column.

$$476 \times 54 \qquad \begin{array}{r} 476 \\ \times\ 54 \\ \hline \end{array}$$

Partial Products

Multiplication problems with more than one digit in the multiplier create **partial products**. Then you add the partial products to get the final answer, the product. Carrying also may be required when multiplying as shown.

$$\begin{array}{r} {}^{1}\ \ \\ 24 \\ \times\ 13 \\ \hline {}_{1}72 \\ 24 \\ \hline 312 \end{array}$$
72 partial product
24 partial product
312 product

Example 1: 546×32

STEP 1. Multiply 546 by 2, multiplying from right to left: $2 \times 6 = 12$. Write a 2 on the first partial product line and carry a 1. Place the 1 over the 4. Next, multiply: $2 \times 4 = 8$; add the 1 carried to the 8 to get 9. Write the 9 to the left of the 2. Next, multiply: $2 \times 5 = 10$. Write 10 to the left of the 9. 1092 is a partial product.

In Step 2, write the second partial product on the line below 1092. Note that you move over one place to the left to start writing this partial product because the 3 you are multiplying by is in the tens' place. (See Section 3.1, Place Value, page 58.)

$$\begin{array}{r} 11 \\ 1 \\ 546 \\ \times\ 32 \\ \hline 1 \\ 1092 \\ 1638 \\ \hline 17{,}472 \end{array}$$

STEP 2. Multiply 546 by 3 (the number to the left of the factor 2), multiplying from right to left: $3 \times 6 = 18$. Write the 8 below the 9 on the first partial product line, and carry the 1. Place the 1 over the 4. Next, multiply: $3 \times 4 = 12$. Add the 1 carried to the 12 to get 13. Write the 3 to the left of the 8, and carry the 1. Next, multiply: $3 \times 5 = 15$. Add the 1 carried to the 15 to get 16. Write 16 to the left of the 3.

STEP 3. Add the partial products.
The answer is 17,472.

Multiplying by Zero

Any number multiplied by 0 equals 0. In a multiplication problem with a 0 (or more than one 0) in the multiplier, write a 0 in the partial product. Then, move to the next digit to the left in the multiplier and continue multiplying as shown in Problem 1.

Problem 1:

$$
\begin{array}{r}
1 \\
52 \\
573 \\
\times 208 \\
\hline
1 \\
4584 \quad \text{partial product} \\
11460 \quad \text{partial product} \\
\hline
119{,}184
\end{array}
$$

Problem 2:

$$
\begin{array}{r}
11 \\
11 \\
456 \\
\times 312 \\
\hline
_2912 \quad \text{partial product} \\
_1456 \quad \text{partial product} \\
1368 \quad \text{partial product} \\
\hline
142{,}272
\end{array}
$$

Problems 1 and 2 both contain three-digit multipliers (208 and 312). However, the multiplier with the zero (208) results in only two partial products. The other multiplier (312) with three nonzero digits results in three partial products.

Example 2: 7,251 × 1,009

STEP 1. Start multiplying by 9. Think, 9 × 1 = 9. Write the
9 on the first partial product line. Next, multiply:
9 × 5 = 45. Write down the 5 and carry the 4.
Next, multiply: 9 × 2 =18; add the 4 carried to
the 18 to get 22. Write down the 2 and carry a
2. Next, multiply: 9 × 7 = 63; add the 2 carried to
the 63 to get 65. Write 65 to the left of the 2.

STEP 2. Move to the next digit to the left of 9 in 1,009. It
is a 0. Multiply 0 × 1 (or actually 0 × 7251) to get
0. On the second partial product line, move a
space to the left, and write a 0 below the 5 in
the tens' place of 65259.

STEP 3. Move left to the next 0. Multiply 0 × 1
(or 0 × 7,251) to get 0. Write a 0 in the second
partial product line to the left of the 0.

STEP 4. Multiply by 1. Think, 1 × 1 = 1. Write 1 below
the 5 in the thousands' place of 65259.
Multiply: 1 × 5 = 5.
Write down the 5. Multiply: 1 × 2 = 2.
Write down the 2. Multiply: 1 × 7 = 7.
Write down the 7.

STEP 5. Add the partial products.
The answer is 7,316,259.

$$
\begin{array}{r}
{\scriptstyle 2\ 4} \\
7{,}251 \\
\times\ 1{,}009 \\
\hline
65\ 259 \\
7\ 251\ 00 \\
\hline
7{,}316{,}259
\end{array}
$$

1.3   Practice Multiplying Whole Numbers

Solve the following problems. See "Step-by-Step Solutions" (page 221) for the answers.

1. 36 × 27	2. 39 × 42	3. 255 × 43	4. 895 × 68
5. 623 × 79	6. 9,173 × 63	7. 4,329 × 73	8. 4,218 × 27
9. 7,516 × 254	10. 784 × 638	11. 71 × 80	12. 62 × 40
13. 31 × 90	14. 471 × 20	15. 891 × 30	16. 710 × 806
17. 123 × 302	18. 1,002 × 123	19. 801 × 497	20. 4,020 × 202

Dividing Whole Numbers
In this section, we will review:
- division terminology
- remainders
- long division
- estimating when dividing

Division Terminology

The terms used in division problems are **dividend** (the number being divided), **divisor** (the number you are dividing by), and **quotient** (the answer). Division problems may be written in either of two formats.

$$\text{divisor} \overline{)\text{dividend}}^{\text{quotient}} \quad \text{or} \quad \text{dividend} \div \text{divisor} = \text{quotient}$$

Division problems that are written horizontally like $192 \div 4$ must be rewritten in this format, $\text{divisor}\overline{)\text{dividend}}^{\text{quotient}}$ before solving. Saying the problem aloud as you write it will help you place the numbers correctly. The problem $192 \div 4$ is read "192 divided by 4". The problem is written $4\overline{)192}$ to solve. To ensure correct answers, be certain to place the terms in the correct position.

Remainders

Division is the inverse (opposite) of multiplication. When you divide by whole numbers the division either works out evenly (has an answer of 0 after the final subtraction) or has a **remainder** (a number left after subtraction).

This problem works out evenly.

$$
\begin{array}{r}
16 \\
3\overline{)48} \\
-3 \\
\hline
18 \\
-18 \\
\hline
0
\end{array}
$$

This problem does not work out evenly, because it has a remainder.

$$
\begin{array}{r}
18\ \text{r.1} \\
2\overline{)37} \\
-2 \\
\hline
17 \\
-16 \\
\hline
1
\end{array}
$$

Long Division

You can perform short-division problems mentally (in your head) and write just the answer. **Long division** refers to the division process in which the steps must be written to find the answer. You need to perform four steps for each digit in the divisor: **divide, multiply, subtract,** and **bring down**. Repeat this sequence until you have completed the problem. Working division problems neatly and placing each number in the correct column are very important. See the example below.

DIVIDE

$$\frac{2}{4\overline{)84}}$$ 8 divided by 4 is 2.

MULTIPLY

$$\frac{2}{4\overline{)84}}$$

8   2 times 4 is 8.

SUBTRACT

$$\frac{2}{4\overline{)84}}$$

$$-8$$

0   8 minus 8 is 0.

BRING DOWN

$$\frac{2}{4\overline{)84}}$$

$$-8$$

04   Bring down the 4. Begin the next step.

Example 1:   84 ÷ 4

STEP 1. **Divide:** 8 ÷ 4 = 2. Write 2 above the 8 in 84.
Multiply: 2 × 4 = 8. Write 8 under the 8.
Subtract: 8 − 8 = 0. Write 0 under the 8.
Bring down the 4.

STEP 2. **Divide:** 4 ÷ 4 = 1. Write 1 above the 4.
Multiply: 1 × 4 = 4. Write 4 under the 4.
Subtract: 4 − 4 = 0. Write 0 under the 4.
Bring Down: All digits have been brought down, so you have finished the problem.
The final subtraction results in 0; therefore, this problem has no remainder.

$$
\begin{array}{r}
21 \\
4\overline{)84} \\
-8 \\
\hline
04 \\
-4 \\
\hline
0
\end{array}
$$

The answer is 21.

Example 2: 2,352 ÷ 5

STEP 1. **Divide:** Because 5 will not go into 2, consider
23. Since 5 will go into 23, 4 times, write a
4 above the 3 in 2,352.
Multiply: 4 × 5 = 20. Write 20 under 23.
Subtract: 23 − 20 = 3. Write 3 under the 0 in 20.
Bring down the 5. Notice that you now have 35.

STEP 2. **Divide:** 35 ÷ 5 = 7. Write 7 above the 5 in 2,352.
Multiply: 5 × 7 = 35. Write 35 under the 35.
Subtract: 35 − 35 = 0.
Bring down the 2.

STEP 3. **Divide:** The 2 cannot be divided by 5, so write
0 above the 2 in the one's place of 2,352.
Multiply: 0 × 5 = 0. Write 0 under the 2.
Subtract: 2 − 0 = 2.
Bring Down: All digits have been brought
down. The number left after the final
subtraction is 2. The remainder 2 is written r.2.

The answer is 470 r.2.

$$
\begin{array}{r}
470 \text{ r.2} \\
5\overline{)2{,}352} \\
-2\,0 \\
\hline
35 \\
-35 \\
\hline
02 \\
-0 \\
\hline
2
\end{array}
$$

Using Estimating When Dividing

Dividing by two- or three-digit whole numbers requires estimating (trial
and error or making an educated guess), then multiplying to see if your
estimate is correct. If your first try is incorrect, adjust your estimate up or
down, and try again.

Example 3:   1,670 ÷ 63

STEP 1. **Divide:** Because 63 will not go into 1, consider 16. Since 63 will not go into 16, consider 167. Think about 167 ÷ 63. Now, estimate: 60 × 3 = 180. However, 180 is too large, so try 2. Think, 60 × 2 = 120. Write the 2 above the 7 in 1,670.
Multiply: 2 × 63 = 126. Write 126 under 167.
Subtract: 167 − 126 = 41.
Bring down the 0. Notice that you now have 410.

STEP 2. **Divide:** Think about 410 ÷ 63. Use an estimate— 6 × 70 = 420. However, 420 is too large, so try 6 × 60 = 360. Write a 6 above the 0 in 1,670.
Multiply: 6 × 3 = 18. Write 8 under the 0 in 410. Carry the 1 and write it above 6 in the divisor, 63. Then multiply: 6 × 6 = 36. 36 + 1 = 37. Write 37 to the left of the 8, so you have 378.
Subtract: 410 − 378 = 32.
Bring down. All digits have been brought down. The 32 left after the final subtraction is the remainder. Write r.32.

The answer is 26 r.32.

```
         26 r.32
  1
63)1,670
   -1 26
     410
    -378
      32
```

Example 4:   38,241 ÷ 607

STEP 1. **Divide:** Because 607 will not go into 382, consider 3,824 and estimate: 600 × 6 = 3,600. Write 6 above the 4 in 38,241.
Multiply: 6 × 607 = 3,642. Write 3642 under 3824.
Subtract: 3824 − 3642 = 182.
Bring down the 1. Notice that you now have 1821.

STEP 2. **Divide:** Use an estimate—600 × 3 = 1,800. Write a 3 above the 1 in 38,241.
Multiply: 3 × 607 = 1,821. Write 1821 under 1821.
Subtract: 1821 − 1821 = 0. Write 0 below 1821.
Bring Down: All digits have been brought down, so you have finished the problem. The final subtraction results in 0; therefore, this problem has no remainder.

The answer is 63.

```
   2          63
   4
607)38,241
   -3642
     1821
    -1821
        0
```

Practice Dividing Whole Numbers

Solve the following problems. Write the answer with a remainder, if needed. See "Step-by-Step Solutions" (page 222) for the answers.

1. $8\overline{)48}$ 2. $7\overline{)49}$ 3. $9\overline{)85}$ 4. $5\overline{)22}$

5. $28\overline{)695}$ 6. $16\overline{)128}$ 7. $20\overline{)305}$ 8. $68\overline{)207}$

9. $17\overline{)340}$ 10. $49\overline{)993}$ 11. $19\overline{)7,603}$ 12. $13\overline{)3,917}$

13. $51\overline{)47,609}$ 14. $95\overline{)19,475}$ 15. $89\overline{)91,002}$ 16. $630\overline{)4,768}$

17. $716\overline{)3,056}$ 18. $502\overline{)98,762}$ 19. $741\overline{)50,612}$ 20. $789\overline{)835,276}$

Solve the following problems. After taking the test, see "Step-by-Step Solutions" (pages 223 to 224) for the answers. And see "1.1 Adding Whole Numbers," "1.2 Subtracting Whole Numbers," "1.3 Multiplying Whole Numbers," and "1.4 Dividing Whole Numbers," if the chapter test indicates you need additional practice.

Section 1.1

1.   7,203
   + 9,097

2.   12,594
   + 6,789

3.   70,698
   + 5,921

4.   5,742
   + 8,706

5.   39,424
   + 65,875

Section 1.2

6.   5,704
   − 892

7.   6,231
   − 1,576

8.   13,452
   − 9,571

9.   75,004
   − 74,989

10.   90,000
   − 71,234

Section 1.3

11.   734
   × 7

12.   576
   × 24

13.   702
   × 30

14.   9,407
   × 609

15.   12,072
   × 1,005

Section 1.4
Write the answer with a remainder, if needed.

16. $26\overline{)175}$

17. $79\overline{)683}$

18. $756\overline{)35,476}$

19. $642\overline{)25,409}$

20. $708\overline{)350,014}$

Fractions

2.0   Pretest for Fractions

Solve the following problems. After taking the test, see "Step-by-Step Solutions" for the answers (pages 225 to 226). Then, see "2.1 Fraction Terminology," "2.2 Multiplying Fractions," "2.3 Dividing Fractions," "2.4 Finding the Least Common Denominator (LCD)," "2.5 Adding Fractions," and "2.6 Subtracting Fractions," for skill explanations.

Section 2.1

1. Change $\dfrac{50}{4}$ to a mixed number. Reduce if necessary.

2. Change $6\dfrac{7}{8}$ to an improper fraction.

Section 2.2

Write answers in reduced form. Change improper fractions to mixed numbers.

3. $\dfrac{4}{7} \times \dfrac{28}{36}$ 4. $5\dfrac{7}{9} \times 3\dfrac{4}{13}$

Section 2.3

Write answers in reduced form. Change improper fractions to mixed numbers.

5. $\dfrac{9}{14} \div \dfrac{3}{21}$ 6. $5\dfrac{3}{5} \div 2\dfrac{6}{25}$

Write answers in reduced form. Change improper fractions to mixed numbers.

7.
$$
\begin{array}{r}
5\frac{3}{5} \\
+\ 7\frac{4}{15} \\
\hline
\end{array}
$$

8. $\dfrac{1}{5} + \dfrac{3}{8} + \dfrac{7}{10}$

Sections 2.4 and 2.6

Write answers in reduced form. Change improper fractions to mixed numbers.

9. $\dfrac{7}{22} - \dfrac{3}{11}$

10.
$$
\begin{array}{r}
14\frac{5}{8} \\
-\ 5\frac{9}{14} \\
\hline
\end{array}
$$

2.1

Fraction Terminology

In this section, we will review:
- fraction terminology
- changing improper fractions to mixed numbers
- changing mixed numbers to improper fractions
- lowest terms and reduced form
- equivalent fractions

Fraction Terminology

A **fraction** is another way of showing division. The division bar shown in fractions is written either horizontally ($-$) or diagonally ($/$). The horizontal division bar ($-$) is used in this book.

New Notation

These four symbols indicate division:

$\div$, $\overline{)}$, **and division bars** $-$ **or** $/$ **which are written horizontally or diagonally.**

A fraction is written in this form: $\dfrac{\textbf{numerator}}{\textbf{denominator}}$.

There are two ways to say a fraction. For example, $\frac{2}{3}$ is read either as two-thirds or 2 out of 3.

Whole numbers also can be written in fraction form. To write a whole number in fraction form, place the whole number over 1. For example, the whole number 5 is written as $\frac{5}{1}$ in fraction form.

A **proper fraction** has a numerator that is smaller than the denominator. For example, $\frac{3}{17}$ is a proper fraction because the numerator 3 is less than the denominator 17.

An **improper fraction** has a numerator that is greater than or equal to the denominator. For example, $\frac{5}{5}$ and $\frac{7}{5}$ are both improper fractions.

A **mixed number** has a whole number part and a fraction part. The mixed number $1\frac{2}{5}$ contains the whole number 1 and the fraction part $\frac{2}{5}$.

Changing Improper Fractions to Mixed Numbers

An improper fraction can be rewritten as a mixed number.

Example 1: Change the improper fraction $\frac{7}{5}$ to a mixed number.

STEP 1. Write the fraction as a division problem. The fraction $\frac{7}{5}$ means 7 divided by 5 or $5\overline{)7}$.

$$\frac{7}{5} = 5\overline{)7}$$

STEP 2. Divide: $5\overline{)7}$. The number 5 goes into 7 one time with a remainder of 2.

$$\begin{array}{r} 1 \\ 5\overline{)7} \\ -5 \\ \hline 2 \end{array}$$

STEP 3. Observe in the division in Step 2 that the number 1 is the whole number part of a mixed number. The remainder 2 indicates that you have only 2 left out of the 5 you would need to be able to divide again.

Therefore, 2 out of 5 is written as $\frac{2}{5}$. The $\frac{2}{5}$ is the fraction part of the mixed number.

The answer is $1\frac{2}{5}$.

$$5 \overline{)\ 7}^{\,1\frac{2}{5}}$$
$$\underline{-\ 5}$$
$$2$$

Changing Mixed Numbers to Improper Fractions

A mixed number can be written as an improper fraction.

Example 2: Change $1\frac{2}{5}$ to an improper fraction.

STEP 1. Multiply the whole number by the fraction's denominator.

$$1 \times 5 = 5$$

STEP 2. Add that product to the numerator of the fraction.

$$5 + 2 = 7$$

STEP 3. Now, 7 becomes the numerator of the improper fraction. The denominator stays the same as in the mixed number, so 5 is the denominator of the improper fraction.

$$\frac{7}{5}$$

The answer is $\frac{7}{5}$.

Your work should look like this on paper.

$$\frac{(1 \times 5) + 2}{5} = \frac{7}{5}$$

Lowest Terms and Reduced Form

A proper fraction or improper fraction is in **reduced form** or written in the **lowest terms** when 1 is the only **common factor** for the numerator and denominator. Reduced form and lowest terms have the same meaning.

A factor that is common to two or more numbers is called a common factor. (See Section 1.3, Terminology, page 6.)

Reducing a Fraction

The numerator and denominator of a fraction can be reduced or divided by the same number, a common factor (except zero), without changing the value of the fraction.

To reduce a fraction, follow these steps:

1. Factor the numerator.
2. Factor the denominator.
3. Cancel a common factor in the numerator and denominator. Any number divided by itself equals 1.
4. Continue to cancel common factors in the numerator and denominator until 1 is the only common factor of the numerator and denominator. It is not necessary to cancel ones, since $1 \div 1 = 1$.

Example 3: Write $\dfrac{5}{13}$ in reduced form.

STEP 1. Factor the numerator.

$$5 = 1 \times 5$$

STEP 2. Factor the denominator.

$$13 = 1 \times 13$$

STEP 3. Cancel common factors.

$$\frac{5}{13} = \frac{1 \times 5}{1 \times 13} = \frac{5}{13}$$

STEP 4. Since 1 is the only common factor of 5 and 13, $\dfrac{5}{13}$ is already in reduced form.

The answer is $\dfrac{5}{13}$.

Your work should look like this on paper.

$$\frac{5}{13} = \frac{1 \times 5}{1 \times 13} = \frac{5}{13}$$

Example 4: Write $\frac{7}{35}$ in reduced form.

STEP 1. Factor the numerator.

$$7 = 1 \times 7$$

STEP 2. Factor the denominator.

$$35 = 5 \times 7$$

STEP 3. Cancel common factors.

$$\frac{7}{35} = \frac{1 \times \overset{1}{\cancel{7}}}{5 \times \cancel{7}_1} = \frac{1}{5}$$

STEP 4. Reducing is complete since 1 is the only common factor of 1 and 5.

The answer is $\frac{1}{5}$.

Your work should look like this $\dfrac{7}{35} = \dfrac{1 \times \overset{1}{\cancel{7}}}{5 \times \cancel{7}_1} = \dfrac{1}{5}$ or the shortcut

method $\dfrac{\overset{1}{\cancel{7}}}{\cancel{35}_5} = \dfrac{1}{5}$.

Example 5: Write $\frac{30}{45}$ in reduced form.

STEP 1. Factor the numerator.

$$30 = 5 \times 6$$

STEP 2. Factor the denominator.

$$45 = 5 \times 9$$

STEP 3. Cancel common factors.

$$\frac{30}{45} = \frac{\overset{1}{\cancel{5}} \times 6}{\cancel{5}_1 \times 9} = \frac{6}{9}$$

STEP 4. Continue to factor since 1 is not the only common factor of 6 and 9.

$$\frac{6}{9} = \frac{2 \times \overset{1}{\cancel{3}}}{3 \times \cancel{3}_{1}} = \frac{2}{3}$$

STEP 5. Reducing is complete since 1 is the only common factor of 2 and 3.

The answer is $\frac{2}{3}$.

Your work should look like this.

$$\frac{30}{45} = \frac{\overset{1}{\cancel{5}} \times 6}{\cancel{5} \times 9} = \frac{6}{9} = \frac{2 \times \overset{1}{\cancel{3}}}{3 \times \cancel{3}_{1}} = \frac{2}{3} \text{ or the shortcut}$$

method $\dfrac{\overset{2}{\cancel{30}}}{\underset{3}{\cancel{45}}} = \dfrac{2}{3}$.

New Notation: In the following examples and solutions in this book, reducing a fraction is shown using the shortcut method.

Equivalent Fractions

Equivalent fractions are fractions that have the same value. You will use equivalent fractions for solving addition and subtraction problems with different denominators.

For example, $\frac{2}{3}$ and $\frac{4}{6}$ are equivalent fractions. If reduced, $\frac{4}{6}$ equals $\frac{2}{3}$. Another example of equivalent fractions is $\frac{1}{2}$ and $\frac{5}{10}$. If reduced, $\frac{5}{10}$ equals $\frac{1}{2}$.

2.1 Practice Fraction Terminology

Solve the following problems. For the answers, see "Step-by-Step Solutions" (pages 226 to 228).

Write these whole numbers as fractions.

1. 28   2. 72

Change these improper fractions to mixed numbers.

3. $\dfrac{16}{3}$ 4. $\dfrac{23}{5}$ 5. $\dfrac{35}{4}$ 6. $\dfrac{61}{8}$ 7. $\dfrac{49}{4}$

Change these mixed numbers to improper fractions.

8. $10\dfrac{1}{3}$ 9. $7\dfrac{5}{8}$ 10. $9\dfrac{1}{2}$ 11. $2\dfrac{9}{10}$ 12. $4\dfrac{5}{12}$

Write each fraction in reduced form.

13. $\dfrac{4}{12}$ 14. $\dfrac{15}{18}$ 15. $\dfrac{6}{30}$ 16. $\dfrac{40}{100}$

Are these pairs equivalent fractions? Answer yes or no.

17. $\dfrac{1}{2}$ $\dfrac{2}{4}$ 18. $\dfrac{9}{11}$ $\dfrac{54}{66}$ 19. $\dfrac{2}{3}$ $\dfrac{9}{21}$ 20. $\dfrac{7}{12}$ $\dfrac{28}{60}$

2.2   Multiplying Fractions

In this section, we will review:
- the steps used to multiply fractions
- greatest common factor (GCF)
- cross canceling

Basic Multiplication Steps

To multiply fractions, follow these basic steps:

1. Write the problem with all terms in fraction form:

$$\frac{\textbf{numerator}}{\textbf{denominator}}$$. Write whole numbers and mixed numbers in fraction form.

2. Multiply the numerators to obtain a new numerator.
3. Multiply the denominators to get a new denominator.

4. Write the answer in fraction form.
5. Write the answer in reduced form.

Example 1: $\dfrac{2}{3} \times \dfrac{5}{7}$

STEP 1. Multiply the numerators. $2 \times 5 = 10$

STEP 2. Multiply the denominators $3 \times 7 = 21$

STEP 3. Write in fraction form. $\dfrac{10}{21}$

STEP 4. $\dfrac{10}{21}$ is in reduced form.

The answer is $\dfrac{10}{21}$.

Your work should look like this on paper. $\dfrac{2}{3} \times \dfrac{5}{7} = \dfrac{10}{21}$

Greatest Common Factor

The **greatest common factor** (GCF) is the largest number that can be divided evenly into two numbers. For example, the GCF of 4 and 8 is 4 since 4 is the largest number that can be divided evenly into 4 and 8. (See Section 2.1, Lowest Terms and Reduced Form, page 20.)

Cross Canceling

Cross canceling is used only when multiplying two or more fractions and is a method for keeping numbers small. The product is in reduced form after completing cross canceling.

The need for cross canceling is determined by looking diagonally at the numerators and denominators of the fractions to be multiplied. Dividing the diagonal numerator and denominator by their GCF is cross canceling. The GCF must be greater than 1 to cross cancel. Note that in Example 1, no cross canceling was necessary since the GCF for both pairs of diagonal numbers was 1.

Example 2: Use cross canceling to solve $\dfrac{3}{8} \times \dfrac{4}{9}$.

STEP 1. Lightly draw an X over the fractions, crossing through the 3 and 9 and through the 8 and 4

so they look like this $\dfrac{3}{8}\diagup\!\!\!\!\diagdown\dfrac{4}{9}$. The

numbers that are diagonal from each other are the ones you will use for cross canceling.

STEP 2. Consider the 3 and 9. Their GCF is 3. Divide both of them by 3 (3 ÷ 3 = 1 and 9 ÷ 3 = 3) . Write 1 above the 3 and 3 below the 9 as shown. Then, consider the 4 and 8. Their GCF is 4 (4 ÷ 4 = 1 and 8 ÷ 4 = 2) . Write 1 above the 4 and 2 below the 8 as shown.

$$\dfrac{\overset{1}{\cancel{3}}}{\underset{2}{\cancel{8}}} \times \dfrac{\overset{1}{\cancel{4}}}{\underset{3}{\cancel{9}}}$$

STEP 3. Multiply the new numerators and denominators.

$$\dfrac{\overset{1}{\cancel{3}}}{\underset{2}{\cancel{8}}} \times \dfrac{\overset{1}{\cancel{4}}}{\underset{3}{\cancel{9}}} = \dfrac{1}{6}$$

The answer is $\dfrac{1}{6}$.

Example 3: $6 \times \dfrac{3}{4}$

STEP 1. Write the 6 in fraction form.

$$\dfrac{6}{1} \times \dfrac{3}{4}$$

STEP 2. Cross cancel.

$$\dfrac{\overset{3}{\cancel{6}}}{1} \times \dfrac{3}{\underset{2}{\cancel{4}}}$$

STEP 3. Multiply.

$$\frac{\overset{3}{\cancel{6}}}{1} \times \frac{3}{\underset{2}{\cancel{4}}} = \frac{9}{2}$$

STEP 4. Write the improper fraction as a mixed
number.

$$\frac{9}{2} = 4\frac{1}{2}$$

The answer is $4\frac{1}{2}$.

Your work should look like this on paper.

$$6 \times \frac{3}{4} = \frac{\overset{3}{\cancel{6}}}{1} \times \frac{3}{\underset{2}{\cancel{4}}} = \frac{9}{2} = 4\frac{1}{2}$$

Example 4: $2\frac{3}{4} \times 1\frac{2}{3}$

STEP 1. Write the mixed numbers
as improper fractions.

$$2\frac{3}{4} = \frac{11}{4} \text{ and } 1\frac{2}{3} = \frac{5}{3}$$

STEP 2. Multiply the numerators and denominators.

$$\frac{11}{4} \times \frac{5}{3} = \frac{55}{12}$$

STEP 3. Write the improper fraction as a mixed
number.

$$\frac{55}{12} = 4\frac{7}{12}$$

The answer is $4\frac{7}{12}$.

Your work should look like this on paper.

$$2\frac{3}{4} \times 1\frac{2}{3} = \frac{11}{4} \times \frac{5}{3} = \frac{55}{12} = 4\frac{7}{12}$$

Example 5: $\dfrac{5}{7} \times \dfrac{9}{10} \times \dfrac{11}{3}$

STEP 1. Consider the numerator 5. The denominators that are diagonal to 5 are 10 and 3. You can only cross cancel with one denominator. The GCF of 5 and 3 is 1, so you cannot cross cancel. The GCF of 5 and 10 is 5. So, cross cancel the 5 and 10.

$$\dfrac{\overset{1}{\cancel{5}}}{7} \times \dfrac{9}{\underset{2}{\cancel{10}}} \times \dfrac{11}{3}$$

STEP 2. Consider the numerator 9. The denominators that are diagonal to 9 are 7 and 3. You can only cross cancel with one denominator. The GCF of 9 and 7 is 1, so you cannot cross cancel. The GCF of 9 and 3 is 3. So, cross cancel the 9 and 3.

$$\dfrac{\overset{1}{\cancel{5}}}{7} \times \dfrac{\overset{3}{\cancel{9}}}{\underset{2}{\cancel{10}}} \times \dfrac{11}{\underset{1}{\cancel{3}}}$$

STEP 3. Consider the numerator 11. The denominators that are diagonal to 11 are now 7 and 2. Since the GCF of 11, 7, and 2 is 1, you cannot cross cancel any numbers.

STEP 4. Look at the numbers that resulted from the cross cancellations. Be sure that none of these numbers have any common factors diagonally or vertically. If there are none, multiply the numerators, then multiply the denominators.

$$\dfrac{\overset{1}{\cancel{5}}}{7} \times \dfrac{\overset{3}{\cancel{9}}}{\underset{2}{\cancel{10}}} \times \dfrac{11}{\underset{1}{\cancel{3}}} = \dfrac{33}{14}$$

STEP 5. Write the improper fraction as a mixed number.

$$\dfrac{33}{14} = 2\dfrac{5}{14}$$

The answer is $2\dfrac{5}{14}$.

Your work should look like this on paper.

$$\dfrac{\overset{1}{\cancel{5}}}{7} \times \dfrac{\overset{3}{\cancel{9}}}{\underset{2}{\cancel{10}}} \times \dfrac{11}{\underset{1}{\cancel{3}}} = \dfrac{33}{14} = 2\dfrac{5}{14}$$

2.2 Practice Multiplying Fractions

Solve the following problems, using cross canceling whenever possible. Write answers in reduced form, and change improper fractions to mixed numbers. See "Step-by-Step Solutions" (pages 228 to 229) for the answers.

1. $\dfrac{3}{4} \times \dfrac{5}{11}$

2. $\dfrac{3}{5} \times \dfrac{4}{7}$

3. $\dfrac{8}{9} \times \dfrac{27}{16}$

4. $\dfrac{8}{9} \times \dfrac{45}{56}$

5. $\dfrac{5}{24} \times \dfrac{18}{15}$

6. $\dfrac{12}{17} \times \dfrac{3}{27}$

7. $\dfrac{2}{11} \times 4$

8. $9 \times \dfrac{7}{36}$

9. $2\dfrac{3}{5} \times \dfrac{9}{11}$

10. $4\dfrac{1}{3} \times 2\dfrac{2}{5}$

11. $4\dfrac{3}{5} \times 1\dfrac{1}{5}$

12. $3\dfrac{5}{6} \times 9$

13. $4\dfrac{2}{5} \times 14\dfrac{2}{9}$

14. $5\dfrac{3}{4} \times 10\dfrac{5}{7}$

15. $7\dfrac{3}{4} \times \dfrac{3}{7}$

16. $5 \times 8\dfrac{3}{4}$

17. $\dfrac{9}{5} \times \dfrac{3}{13} \times \dfrac{10}{27}$

18. $\dfrac{10}{13} \times \dfrac{26}{15} \times \dfrac{2}{3}$

19. $\dfrac{4}{5} \times \dfrac{15}{44} \times 4$

20. $\dfrac{3}{7} \times \dfrac{4}{10} \times \dfrac{28}{18}$

Dividing Fractions

In this section, we will review:
- the steps used to divide fractions
- reciprocals

Basic Division Steps

To divide fractions, follow these basic steps:

1. Write the problem with all terms in fraction form:

    $$\frac{\text{numerator}}{\text{denominator}}.$$ Write whole numbers and mixed numbers

    in fraction form.
2. Change the division sign to a multiplication sign.
3. Write the reciprocal of the second fraction.
4. Cross cancel if possible (see page 25).
5. Multiply the numerators and denominators.
6. Write the answer in reduced form.

Changing Signs

Changing the division sign ($\div$) to a multiplication sign ($\times$) means just what it says.

For instance, change $\dfrac{5}{8} \div \dfrac{7}{11}$ to $\dfrac{5}{8} \times \dfrac{11}{7}$.

Reciprocals

To find the **reciprocal** of the fraction, invert or flip the fraction. For instance:

- to find the reciprocal of $\dfrac{3}{4}$, simply invert: $\dfrac{4}{3}$

- to find the reciprocal of 5, first write 5 in fraction form: $\dfrac{5}{1}$, then invert: $\dfrac{1}{5}$

- to find the reciprocal of $1\dfrac{2}{3}$, first write $1\dfrac{2}{3}$ as an improper fraction: $\dfrac{5}{3}$, then invert: $\dfrac{3}{5}$

Example 1: $\dfrac{3}{4} \div \dfrac{2}{3}$

STEP 1. Make no change in the terms because both terms are in fraction form.

$$\dfrac{3}{4} \div \dfrac{2}{3}$$

STEP 2. Change the division sign to a multiplication sign.

$$\dfrac{3}{4} \times$$

STEP 3. Write the reciprocal of the second fraction.

The reciprocal of $\dfrac{2}{3}$ is $\dfrac{3}{2}$.

$$\dfrac{3}{4} \times \dfrac{3}{2}$$

STEP 4. Skip cross canceling because 3 and 2 as well as 4 and 3 have no common factors.

STEP 5. Multiply the numerators and denominators.

$$\dfrac{3}{4} \times \dfrac{3}{2} = \dfrac{9}{8}$$

STEP 6. Write the improper fraction as a mixed number.

$$\dfrac{9}{8} = 1\dfrac{1}{8}$$

The answer is $1\dfrac{1}{8}$.

Your work should look like this on paper.

$$\dfrac{3}{4} \div \dfrac{2}{3} = \dfrac{3}{4} \times \dfrac{3}{2} = \dfrac{9}{8} = 1\dfrac{1}{8}$$

Example 2: $\dfrac{5}{8} \div 5$

STEP 1. Write 5 in fraction form: $\dfrac{5}{1}$.

$$\dfrac{5}{8} \div \dfrac{5}{1}$$

STEP 2. Change the division sign to a multiplication sign.

$$\dfrac{5}{8} \times$$

STEP 3. Observe that the reciprocal of $\dfrac{5}{1}$ is $\dfrac{1}{5}$.

$$\dfrac{5}{8} \times \dfrac{1}{5}$$

STEP 4. Cross cancel the 5s. Their GCF is 5.

$$\dfrac{\overset{1}{\cancel{5}}}{8} \times \dfrac{1}{\underset{1}{\cancel{5}}}$$

STEP 5. Multiply the numerators and denominators.

$$\dfrac{\overset{1}{\cancel{5}}}{8} \times \dfrac{1}{\underset{1}{\cancel{5}}} = \dfrac{1}{8}$$

STEP 6. Make no changes to the fraction; it is in its reduced form: $\dfrac{1}{8}$.

The answer is $\dfrac{1}{8}$.

Your work should look like this on paper.

$$\dfrac{5}{8} \div 5 = \dfrac{5}{8} \div \dfrac{5}{1} = \dfrac{\overset{1}{\cancel{5}}}{8} \times \dfrac{1}{\underset{1}{\cancel{5}}} = \dfrac{1}{8}$$

Example 3: $8\frac{4}{5} \div 4\frac{8}{15}$

STEP 1. Change the mixed numbers to improper fractions.

$$\frac{44}{5} \div \frac{68}{15}$$

STEP 2. Change the division sign to a multiplication sign.

$$\frac{44}{5} \times \frac{15}{68}$$

STEP 3. Observe that the reciprocal of $\frac{68}{15}$ is $\frac{15}{68}$.

STEP 4. Cross cancel the 44 and the 68. Their GCF is 4. The 5 and the 15 have a GCF of 5.

$$\frac{\overset{11}{\cancel{44}}}{\underset{1}{\cancel{5}}} \times \frac{\overset{3}{\cancel{15}}}{\underset{17}{\cancel{68}}}$$

STEP 5. Multiply the numerators and denominators.

$$\frac{\overset{11}{\cancel{44}}}{\underset{1}{\cancel{5}}} \times \frac{\overset{3}{\cancel{15}}}{\underset{17}{\cancel{68}}} = \frac{33}{17}$$

STEP 6. Write the improper fraction as a mixed number.

$$\frac{33}{17} = 1\frac{16}{17}$$

The answer is $1\frac{16}{17}$.

Your work should look like this on paper.

$$8\frac{4}{5} \div 4\frac{8}{15} = \frac{44}{5} \div \frac{68}{15} = \frac{\overset{11}{\cancel{44}}}{\underset{1}{\cancel{5}}} \times \frac{\overset{3}{\cancel{15}}}{\underset{17}{\cancel{68}}} = \frac{33}{17} = 1\frac{16}{17}$$

Rules for Dividing with Zero

Two rules govern division with zero.

Rule 1. Zero divided by any number equals 0: $\dfrac{0}{\textbf{any number}} = \textbf{0}$.

For example, $\dfrac{\textbf{0}}{\textbf{2}} = \textbf{0}$.

Rule 2. Zero divided by any number is undefined (or has no solution):

$$\frac{\textbf{any number}}{\textbf{0}} = \textbf{undefined or no solution.}$$

For example, $\dfrac{\textbf{5}}{\textbf{0}} = \textbf{undefined}$.

2.3 Practice Dividing Fractions

Solve the following problems. Change division to multiplication, and cross cancel if possible. Multiply and reduce if needed. See "Step-by-Step Solutions" (pages 229 to 231) for the answers.

1. $\dfrac{7}{10} \div \dfrac{14}{25}$
2. $\dfrac{2}{5} \div \dfrac{5}{7}$
3. $\dfrac{7}{8} \div \dfrac{2}{3}$

4. $\dfrac{2}{9} \div \dfrac{1}{6}$
5. $12 \div \dfrac{3}{4}$
6. $\dfrac{5}{6} \div 18$

7. $0 \div \dfrac{5}{16}$
8. $1 \div \dfrac{3}{7}$
9. $6\dfrac{3}{16} \div 1\dfrac{5}{8}$

10. $4\dfrac{2}{3} \div \dfrac{7}{27}$
11. $6\dfrac{2}{5} \div 3$
12. $2\dfrac{1}{3} \div 6\dfrac{5}{8}$

13. $2\dfrac{3}{8} \div 5\dfrac{3}{7}$
14. $\dfrac{24}{29} \div 0$
15. $2\dfrac{1}{15} \div 3\dfrac{1}{3}$

16. $6\frac{1}{2} \div 2\frac{3}{4}$ 17. $12\frac{1}{2} \div 5\frac{5}{6}$ 18. $4\frac{3}{5} \div 10$

19. $6\frac{3}{4} \div 3\frac{1}{2}$ 20. $4\frac{5}{9} \div 2\frac{1}{3}$

| 2.4 | **Finding the Least Common Denominator (LCD)** |

In this section, we will review:
- least common denominator
- prime numbers

Terminology

The smallest whole number into which several other whole numbers will divide evenly is called the **least common multiple**. When working with fractions, the least common multiple is referred to as the **least common denominator (LCD)**. You will need the least common denominator when adding or subtracting fractions with unlike denominators.

Use **prime numbers** to find the least common denominator. A **prime number** is a whole number greater than 1 that can be divided evenly only by 1 and itself. These are the prime numbers less than 50: 2, 3, 5, 7, 11, 13, 17, 19, 23, 29, 31, 37, 41, 43, 47

The examples illustrate the step-by-step process to find the LCD. Here are general pointers to keep in mind.

- Look at the denominators of the fractions and recall their factors.
- If the denominators have no common factors, multiply them together to get the LCD.
- If the denominators have a common factor, look at the list of primes and determine the smallest prime number that can be divided into the denominators evenly (without a remainder). Begin dividing with that number. You must divide by only prime numbers.
- Continue dividing by the same prime until it no longer divides evenly. Then move up the list of primes to see if a larger prime number is a factor of both numbers.

- The division process is complete when your bottom row of quotients has no common prime factor.
- If there are three denominators, the prime number must be a factor of at least two of the denominators. The third denominator is not divided, it is just moved down to the next row.
- Remember to multiply the prime numbers along the left side of the L shape and the numbers in the bottom row of quotients to find the LCD.

Example 1: Find the LCD for $\dfrac{5}{6}$ and $\dfrac{7}{15}$.

STEP 1. Observe that the denominators are 6 and 15.

STEP 2. Write 6 and 15 next to each other. Draw an L around them.

$$\lfloor 6 \quad 15$$

STEP 3. Find their least common prime factor. The 6 and 15 are both divisible by 3, so place a 3 to the left of the L as shown.

$$3\,\lfloor 6 \quad 15$$

STEP 4. Next, divide 6 and 15 by 3; $6 \div 3 = 2$ and $15 \div 3 = 5$. Write the quotients below 6 and 15 as shown.

$$3\,\lfloor 6 \quad 15$$
$$\quad\;\; 2 \quad 5$$

STEP 5. Since the numbers in the row (2 and 5) have no common factors, stop dividing. Circle the number to the left of the L and the numbers below the L as shown.

$$\boxed{3}\,\lfloor 6 \quad 15$$
$$\quad\;\; \boxed{2 \quad 5}$$

STEP 6. Multiply the circled numbers.

$$3 \cdot 2 \cdot 5 = 30$$

The answer is 30.

New Notation

Both • and × mean to multiply.

Example 2: Find the LCD for $\frac{3}{4}$ and $\frac{7}{9}$.

STEP 1. Observe that the denominators are 4 and 9.

STEP 2. Write 4 and 9 next to each other. Draw an L around them.

$\lfloor 4 \quad 9$

STEP 3. Notice that the numbers 4 and 9 have no common prime factors.

Step 4. Multiply them together.

$4 \cdot 9 = 36$

The answer is 36.

Example 3: You are given the denominators 12 and 42. Find the least common denominator.

STEP 1. Write 12 and 42 next to each other. Draw an L around them like this:

$\lfloor 12 \quad 42$

STEP 2. Find their least common prime factor: The 12 and 42 are both divisible by 2, so place a 2 to the left of the L and divide as shown.

$2 \lfloor \underline{12 \quad 42}$
$\quad\; 6 \quad 21$

STEP 3. Then write the resulting 6 and 21 with an L around them like this. The 6 and 21 are both divisible by 3. Write 3 to the left of the L and divide.

$2 \lfloor \underline{12 \quad 42}$
$3 \lfloor \underline{6 \quad 21}$
$\quad\; 2 \quad 7$

STEP 4. Stop dividing since the numbers 2 and 7 have no common prime factors. Circle the factors on the left of the L and the numbers below the L as shown.

$2 \lfloor \underline{12 \quad 42}$
$3 \lfloor \underline{6 \quad 21}$
$\quad\; 2 \quad 7$

STEP 5. Multiply the circled numbers:

$2 \cdot 3 \cdot 2 \cdot 7 = 84$

The answer is 84.

You can use the same method with one variation to find the LCD of three fractions. The variation is that at least two of the three numbers in a row must have a common factor to proceed. Simply bring down to the next row with the other quotients the number that is not divisible by the common factor.

Example 4: $\dfrac{3}{16} + \dfrac{7}{20} + \dfrac{17}{30}$

STEP 1. Observe that the denominators are 16, 20, and 30. Write the denominators next to each and draw the L around them.

$$\underline{16 \quad 20 \quad 30}$$

STEP 2. Observe that the least common prime factor of 16, 20, and 30 is 2. Divide them by 2.

$$2\underline{\,|\,16 \quad 20 \quad 30}$$
$$8 \quad 10 \quad 15$$

STEP 3. Notice that the resulting row contains 8, 10, and 15. There is no common prime factor for those three numbers. However, two of the numbers, 8 and 10, have a common prime factor of 2. Therefore, write the 2 to the left of the L and divide. Write 4 and 5 under the 8 and 10 as shown. The 15 cannot be divided by 2, so bring it down as shown.

$$2\underline{\,|\,16 \quad 20 \quad 30}$$
$$2\underline{\,|\,\;8 \quad 10 \quad 15}$$
$$\qquad\qquad\qquad\downarrow$$
$$4 \quad 5 \quad 15$$

STEP 4. The resulting row contains 4, 5, and 15. There is no common prime factor for 4, 5, and 15. However, two of the numbers, 5 and 15, have a common prime factor of 5.

Therefore, write the 5 to the left of the L and divide. Place the 1 and 3 below the 5 and 15 as shown. Because 4 cannot be divided by 5, bring it down as shown.

$$2\underline{\,|\,16 \quad 20 \quad 30}$$
$$2\underline{\,|\,\;8 \quad 10 \quad 15}$$
$$\qquad\qquad\qquad\downarrow$$
$$5\;|\;4 \quad 5 \quad 15$$
$$\downarrow$$
$$4 \quad 1 \quad 3$$

STEP 5. Stop dividing since the numbers in the row (4, 1, and 3) have no common factors. Circle the factors on the left of the L and the numbers below the L as shown.

$$2\underline{\,|\,16 \quad 20 \quad 30}$$
$$2\underline{\,|\,\;8 \quad 10 \quad 15}$$
$$\qquad\qquad\qquad\downarrow$$
$$5\;|\;4 \quad 5 \quad 15$$
$$\downarrow$$
$$4 \quad 1 \quad 3$$

STEP 6. Multiply the circled numbers:

$$2 \cdot 2 \cdot 5 \cdot 4 \cdot 1 \cdot 3 = 240$$

The answer is 240.

2.4 Practice Finding the Least Common Denominator

Solve the following problems. For the answers, see "Step-by-Step Solutions" (pages 231 to 233).
Find the least common multiple for the following pairs of numbers.

1. 12 and 24

2. 20 and 30

3. 40 and 10

4. 8 and 18

5. 42 and 35

6. 12 and 8

7. 40 and 25

8. 40 and 50

9. 32 and 40

10. 30 and 36

Find the LCD for each of the following fractions.

11. $\dfrac{8}{35}$ and $\dfrac{11}{14}$

12. $\dfrac{4}{33}$ and $\dfrac{5}{22}$

13. $\dfrac{7}{15}$ and $\dfrac{19}{36}$

14. $\dfrac{5}{21}$ and $\dfrac{4}{9}$

15. $\dfrac{5}{18}$ and $\dfrac{17}{24}$

16. $\dfrac{7}{25}$ and $\dfrac{13}{50}$

17. $\dfrac{1}{3}$ and $\dfrac{5}{6}$ and $\dfrac{7}{9}$

18. $\dfrac{2}{3}$ and $\dfrac{1}{5}$ and $\dfrac{7}{12}$

19. $\dfrac{5}{16}$ and $\dfrac{11}{18}$ and $\dfrac{17}{24}$

20. $\dfrac{3}{4}$ and $\dfrac{5}{6}$ and $\dfrac{7}{8}$

Adding Fractions

In this section, we will review:
- adding fractions
- forming equivalent fractions

Addition Basics

To add fractions, the denominators must be the same. But, you also will encounter these situations:
- different denominators
- one denominator that is a multiple of the other
- mixed numbers

Same Denominators

To add fractions with the same denominators, follow these basic steps:

1. Add the numerators. The denominator stays the same.
2. Reduce the answer if needed.

Example 1: $\dfrac{1}{7} + \dfrac{3}{7}$

STEP 1. Add the numerators. The denominator stays the same.

$$\frac{1+3}{7} = \frac{4}{7}$$

STEP 2. Observe that the fraction $\dfrac{4}{7}$ is in reduced form.

The answer is $\dfrac{4}{7}$.

Your work should look like this on paper.

$$\frac{1}{7} + \frac{3}{7} = \frac{4}{7}$$

Different Denominators

To add fractions with different denominators, follow these basic steps:

1. Find the LCD. (See Section 2.4 "Finding the Least Common Denominator," page 35.)
2. Write equivalent fractions. (See Section 2.1 "Fraction Terminology," page 18.)
3. Add the numerators. The denominator stays the same.
4. Reduce the answer if needed.

Forming Equivalent Fractions

When you multiply a fraction by 1 or in this case, a fraction that equals 1 (like, $\frac{2}{2}$), the value of the fraction remains the same. The resulting fraction is an equivalent fraction. An equivalent fraction when reduced equals the original fraction. Forming equivalent fractions makes the denominators of different fractions the same, thus making it possible to add. To form equivalent fractions follow these steps:

1. Find the LCD for the denominators.
2. Multiply one or both fractions by a fractional form of 1, like, $\frac{5}{5}$, so equivalent fractions formed have the same denominator.

Example 2: $\quad \frac{1}{3} + \frac{5}{8}$

STEP 1. Observe that the LCD of 3 and 8 is 24 since they have no common factors.

$$3 \cdot 8 = 24$$
The LCD is 24.

STEP 2. Form equivalent fractions. Multiply $\frac{1}{3}$ by $\frac{8}{8}$ to form an equivalent fraction that has a denominator of 24. And multiply $\frac{5}{8}$ by $\frac{3}{3}$ to form an equivalent fraction that has a denominator of 24.

$$\frac{1}{3} \cdot \frac{8}{8} = \frac{8}{24}$$
$$+ \frac{5}{8} \cdot \frac{3}{3} = \frac{15}{24}$$

STEP 3. Add the equivalent fractions.

$$\frac{1}{3} \cdot \frac{8}{8} = \frac{8}{24}$$
$$+ \frac{5}{8} \cdot \frac{3}{3} = \frac{15}{24}$$
$$\frac{23}{24}$$

The answer is $\frac{23}{24}$.

Example 3: $\dfrac{1}{12} + \dfrac{3}{20}$

STEP 1. Find the LCD of 12 and 20.

$$
\begin{array}{c|cc}
2 & 12 & 20 \\
2 & 6 & 10 \\
\hline
 & 3 & 5
\end{array}
$$

$$2 \cdot 2 \cdot 3 \cdot 5 = 60$$

The LCD is 60.

STEP 2. Form equivalent fractions with a denominator of 60.

$$\dfrac{1}{12} \cdot \dfrac{5}{5} = \dfrac{5}{60}$$
$$+ \dfrac{3}{20} \cdot \dfrac{3}{3} = \dfrac{9}{60}$$

STEP 3. Add the numerators. The denominator stays the same.

$$\dfrac{1}{12} \cdot \dfrac{5}{5} = \dfrac{5}{60}$$
$$+ \dfrac{3}{20} \cdot \dfrac{3}{3} = \dfrac{9}{60}$$

STEP 4. Reduce the fraction.

$$\dfrac{14^{7}}{60_{30}} = \dfrac{7}{30}$$

The answer is $\dfrac{7}{30}$.

One Denominator Is A Multiple of the Other

To add fractions in which one fraction's denominator is a multiple of the other's denominator—such as 2 and 4; 6 and 24; or 7 and 56—follow these steps:

1. Find the LCD. The LCD in this type of problem is the larger of the two numbers.
2. Form an equivalent fraction.
3. Add the numerators. The denominators remain the same.
4. Reduce the fraction if needed.

Example 4: $\dfrac{3}{4} + \dfrac{7}{16}$

STEP 1. Find the LCD: Because 16 is a multiple of 4, 16 is the LCD.

The LCD is 16.

STEP 2. Form equivalent fractions with a denominator of 16. Because 16 is the LCD, $\dfrac{7}{16}$ remains the same.

$$\dfrac{3}{4} \cdot \dfrac{4}{4} = \dfrac{12}{16}$$
$$+\dfrac{7}{16} \qquad = \dfrac{7}{16}$$

STEP 3. Add the numerators. The denominator stays the same.

$$\dfrac{3}{4} \cdot \dfrac{4}{4} = \dfrac{12}{16}$$
$$+\dfrac{7}{16} \qquad = \dfrac{7}{16}$$
$$\dfrac{19}{16}$$

STEP 4. Change the improper fraction to a mixed number.

$$\dfrac{19}{16} = 1\dfrac{3}{16}$$

The answer is $1\dfrac{3}{16}$.

Your work should look like this on paper.

$$\dfrac{3}{4} \cdot \dfrac{4}{4} = \dfrac{12}{16}$$
$$+\dfrac{7}{16} \qquad = \dfrac{7}{16}$$
$$\dfrac{19}{16} = 1\dfrac{3}{16}$$

Mixed Numbers

To add mixed numbers like $3\frac{2}{3}$ and $4\frac{4}{8}$, follow these steps:

1. Find the LCD, if the fractions have different denominators.
2. Form equivalent fractions, if needed.
3. Add the fractions' numerators. The denominators remain the same. Then add the whole number parts of the mixed number(s).
4. Change improper fractions to a mixed number, if needed.
5. Reduce the fraction part of the mixed number, if needed.
6. Add the mixed number to the whole number sum.

Example 5: $3\frac{2}{3} + 4\frac{6}{7}$

STEP 1. Find the LCD. The 3 and 7 have no common factors, so the LCD is 21.

$$3 \cdot 7 = 21$$
$$\text{The LCD is 21.}$$

STEP 2. Form equivalent fractions.

$$3\frac{2}{3} \cdot \frac{7}{7} = 3\frac{14}{21}$$
$$+\;4\frac{6}{7} \cdot \frac{3}{3} = 4\frac{18}{21}$$

STEP 3. Add the numerators. The denominators remain the same. Then add the whole numbers.

$$3\frac{2}{3} \cdot \frac{7}{7} = 3\frac{14}{21}$$
$$+\;4\frac{6}{7} \cdot \frac{3}{3} = 4\frac{18}{21}$$
$$7\frac{32}{21}$$

STEP 4. Change the improper fraction to a mixed number.

$$\frac{32}{21} = 1\frac{11}{21}$$

STEP 5. Notice that the fraction part, $\frac{11}{21}$ cannot be reduced.

STEP 6. Add 7, the sum of the whole number part to the mixed number $1\frac{11}{21}$.

$$7 + 1\frac{11}{21} = 8\frac{11}{21}$$

The answer is $8\frac{11}{21}$.

Your work should look like this on paper.

$$3\frac{2}{3} \cdot \frac{7}{7} = 3\frac{14}{21}$$
$$+ 4\frac{6}{7} \cdot \frac{3}{3} = + 4\frac{18}{21}$$
$$\overline{\hspace{3cm}}$$
$$7\frac{32}{21} = 7 + 1\frac{11}{21} = 8\frac{11}{21}$$

2.5 Practice Adding Fractions

Solve the following problems. For the answers, see "Step-by-Step Solutions" (pages 233 to 236).
Reduce if needed.

1.
$$\frac{1}{5}$$
$$+ \frac{3}{5}$$

2.
$$\frac{4}{7}$$
$$+ \frac{3}{14}$$

3.
$$\frac{9}{11}$$
$$+ \frac{4}{5}$$

4.
$$7\frac{1}{8}$$
$$+ 2\frac{5}{8}$$

5.
$$5\frac{4}{5}$$
$$+ 3\frac{3}{10}$$

6.
$$1\frac{5}{6}$$
$$+ \frac{7}{8}$$

7.
$$4\frac{1}{3}$$
$$+ 2\frac{1}{4}$$

8.
$$47\frac{3}{10}$$
$$+ 26\frac{5}{8}$$

Continued

9. $34\frac{1}{20}$
$+ 45\frac{8}{15}$

10. $25\frac{3}{14}$
$+ 58\frac{1}{7}$

11. $2\frac{5}{33}$
$+ \frac{3}{11}$

12. $5\frac{3}{10}$
$+ 2\frac{1}{14}$

13. $8\frac{2}{9}$
$+ 4\frac{3}{4}$

14. $4\frac{1}{6}$
$+ 13\frac{9}{10}$

15. $6\frac{4}{9}$
$+ 12\frac{1}{15}$

16. $7\frac{3}{5}$
$+ 2\frac{1}{8}$

17. $\frac{1}{3}$
$\frac{1}{8}$
$+ \frac{1}{6}$

18. $\frac{1}{12}$
$\frac{3}{14}$
$+ \frac{4}{21}$

19. $3\frac{1}{20} + 7\frac{1}{15} + 2\frac{3}{10}$

20. $27\frac{2}{3} + 30\frac{5}{8} + 31\frac{5}{6}$

2.6   **Subtracting Fractions**

In this section, we will review:
• subtracting fractions
• subtracting mixed numbers
• borrowing with mixed numbers

Subtraction Basics

To subtract fractions, the denominators must be the same. First, we will show you how to subtract fractions when the denominators are the same, then we will show you what to do when they are different.

Same Denominators

To subtract fractions with the same denominators, follow these basic steps:

1. Subtract the numerators in the fraction part. Write the difference (answer) over the denominator.
2. Subtract the whole number part, if necessary.
3. Reduce, if needed.

Example 1: $\dfrac{5}{9} - \dfrac{3}{9}$

STEP 1. Subtract the numerators. Write the difference over the denominator.

$$\dfrac{5-3}{9}$$

STEP 2. Observe that there is no whole number part to subtract.

STEP 3. Notice that the answer is in reduced form.

$$\dfrac{5}{9} - \dfrac{3}{9} = \dfrac{2}{9}$$

The answer is $\dfrac{2}{9}$.

Example 2: $4\dfrac{5}{37} - 2\dfrac{4}{37}$

STEP 1. Subtract the numerators in the fraction part.

5 − 4 = 1. Write the difference over the denominator to show $\dfrac{1}{37}$.

STEP 2. Subtract the whole numbers: 4 − 2 = 2. Now you have $2\dfrac{1}{37}$.

STEP 3. Notice that the answer is in reduced form.

$$\begin{array}{r} 4\dfrac{5}{37} \\ -\,2\dfrac{4}{37} \\ \hline 2\dfrac{1}{37} \end{array}$$

The answer is $2\dfrac{1}{37}$.

Different Denominators

To subtract fractions with different denominators, follow these steps:

1. Find the LCD.
2. Change the fractions to equivalent fractions.
3. Subtract the numerators, if possible. The numerator in the top term must be larger than the numerator in the bottom term. Write the difference (answer) over the denominator.
4. Subtract the whole numbers, if needed.
5. Reduce, if needed.

Example 3: $\dfrac{5}{6} - \dfrac{3}{4}$

STEP 1. Find the least common denominator of 6 and 4.

$$2\,|\,\underline{6\quad 4}$$
$$3\quad 2$$

$$2 \cdot 3 \cdot 2 = 12$$
The LCD is 12.

STEP 2. Form equivalent fractions.

$$\frac{5}{6} \cdot \frac{2}{2} = \frac{10}{12} \text{ and } \frac{3}{4} \cdot \frac{3}{3} = \frac{9}{12}$$

STEP 3. Subtract the numerators in the fraction part.

$10 - 9 = 1$. Write the difference over the denominator to show $\dfrac{1}{12}$.

STEP 4. Observe that there are no whole numbers to subtract.

$$\frac{5}{6} \cdot \frac{2}{2} = \frac{10}{12}$$
$$-\frac{3}{4} \cdot \frac{3}{3} = -\frac{9}{12}$$
$$\frac{1}{12}$$

STEP 5. Notice that the answer is in reduced form.

The answer is $\dfrac{1}{12}$.

Example 4: $7\frac{5}{6} - 4\frac{3}{14}$

STEP 1. Find the least common denominator of 6 and 14.

$$2 \underline{|\; 6 \quad 14}$$
$$ \underline{3 \quad 7}$$

$$2 \cdot 3 \cdot 7 = 42$$

The LCD is 42.

STEP 2. Form equivalent fractions.

$$\frac{5}{6} \cdot \frac{7}{7} = \frac{35}{42} \text{ and } \frac{3}{14} \cdot \frac{3}{3} = \frac{9}{42}$$

STEP 3. Subtract the numerators in the fraction part. $35 - 9 = 26$. Write the difference over the denominator.

$$7\frac{5}{6} \cdot \frac{7}{7} = 7\frac{35}{42}$$
$$-4\frac{3}{14} \cdot \frac{3}{3} = -4\frac{9}{42}$$

STEP 4. Subtract the whole numbers: $7 - 4 = 3$. Now you have 3.

$$3\frac{\overset{13}{\cancel{26}}}{\underset{21}{\cancel{42}}} = 3\frac{13}{21}$$

STEP 5. Reduce $\frac{26}{42}$ to $\frac{13}{21}$.

The answer is $3\frac{13}{21}$.

Borrowing

Borrowing from the whole number of a mixed number is required when the numerator of the bottom fraction is larger than the numerator of the top fraction.

For example, in the problem $\begin{array}{r} 3\frac{2}{9} \\ -\ \frac{5}{9} \\ \hline \end{array}$, you cannot subtract $\frac{5}{9}$ from $\frac{2}{9}$. So you must borrow 1 from the 3. Since $1 = \frac{9}{9}$, the whole number 3 is rewritten as $2\frac{9}{9}$ and then added to the fractional part of the top number, $\frac{2}{9}$. This is shown as: $3\frac{2}{9} = \overset{2\frac{9}{9}}{\cancel{3}\frac{2}{9}} = 2\frac{9}{9} + \frac{2}{9} = 2\frac{11}{9}$. Now it is possible to subtract $\frac{5}{9}$.

Tip: You can use a shortcut for rewriting mixed numbers when borrowing is needed.

STEP 1. Subtract 1 from the whole number.

STEP 2. Add the numerator and denominator in the fraction part.

STEP 3. Place that sum over the denominator.

STEP 4. Write the lowered whole number and the new improper fraction.

Example 5: Use the shortcut to rewrite $5\frac{7}{16}$ so that you can borrow.

STEP 1. Subtract 1 from the whole number. $5 - 1 = 4$

STEP 2. Add the numerator and denominator. $7 + 16 = 23$

STEP 3. Place that sum over the denominator. $\frac{23}{16}$

STEP 4: Write the lowered whole number and the new improper fraction. $4\frac{23}{16}$

The answer is $4\frac{23}{16}$.

Example 6: $7\dfrac{1}{8} - \dfrac{5}{8}$

STEP 1. Consider that you cannot subtract $\dfrac{5}{8}$

from $\dfrac{1}{8}$. Borrow and rewrite $7\dfrac{1}{8}$ as $6\dfrac{9}{8}$.

STEP 2. Subtract the numerators in the fraction

part $(9 - 5 = 4)$. Write the difference

over the denominator to show $\dfrac{4}{8}$.

STEP 3. Bring down the 6. Now you have $6\dfrac{4}{8}$.

STEP 4. Reduce $6\dfrac{4}{8}$ to $6\dfrac{1}{2}$.

$$7\dfrac{1}{8} = 6\dfrac{9}{8}$$
$$-\dfrac{5}{8} = -\dfrac{5}{8}$$
$$6\dfrac{\cancel{4}^{1}}{\cancel{8}_{2}} = 6\dfrac{1}{2}$$

The answer is $6\dfrac{1}{2}$.

Example 7: $16\dfrac{5}{8} - 13\dfrac{11}{12}$

STEP 1. Find the least common denominator
of 8 and 12.

$$\begin{array}{r|cc} 2 & 8 & 12 \\ 2 & 4 & 6 \\ \hline & 2 & 3 \end{array}$$

$$2 \cdot 2 \cdot 2 \cdot 3 = 24$$
The LCD is 24.

STEP 2. Form equivalent fractions.

$$\dfrac{5}{8} \cdot \dfrac{3}{3} = \dfrac{15}{24} \text{ and } \dfrac{11}{12} \cdot \dfrac{2}{2} = \dfrac{22}{24}$$

STEP 3. Consider that you cannot subtract $\frac{22}{24}$ from

$\frac{15}{24}$. Borrow and rewrite $16\frac{15}{24}$ as $15\frac{39}{24}$.

$$16\frac{5}{8} = 16\frac{5}{8} \cdot \frac{3}{3} = 16\frac{15}{24} = 15\frac{39}{24}$$

$$-13\frac{11}{12} = -13\frac{11}{12} \cdot \frac{2}{2} = -13\frac{22}{24} = -13\frac{22}{24}$$

STEP 4. Subtract the numerators in the fraction part.

$2\frac{17}{24}$

39 − 22 = 17 . Write the difference over the

denominator to show $\frac{17}{24}$. Subtract the

whole numbers. 15 − 13 = 2.

STEP 5. Notice that the answer is in reduced form.

The answer is $2\frac{17}{24}$.

2.6 Practice Subtracting Fractions

Solve the following problems. For the answers, see "Step-by-Step Solutions" (pages 236 to 238).
Borrow if necessary. Reduce all answers.

1. $\frac{3}{4} - \frac{1}{4}$ 2. $\frac{84}{89} - \frac{32}{89}$ 3. $\frac{37}{20} - \frac{4}{5}$

4. $\begin{array}{r} \frac{3}{9} \\ -\ \frac{1}{7} \\ \hline \end{array}$ 5. $\begin{array}{r} \frac{9}{50} \\ -\ \frac{2}{25} \\ \hline \end{array}$ 6. $\begin{array}{r} \frac{5}{12} \\ -\ \frac{7}{30} \\ \hline \end{array}$

7. $\begin{array}{r} \frac{11}{24} \\ -\ \frac{0}{4} \\ \hline \end{array}$ 8. $\begin{array}{r} 7\frac{11}{12} \\ -\ 3\frac{5}{12} \\ \hline \end{array}$ 9. $\begin{array}{r} 6\frac{7}{8} \\ -\ 4\frac{3}{8} \\ \hline \end{array}$

10.
$$18\frac{5}{6}$$
$$-\ 10\frac{1}{4}$$

11.
$$10\frac{3}{8}$$
$$-\ 1\frac{3}{4}$$

12.
$$18\frac{1}{6}$$
$$-\ 10\frac{3}{4}$$

13.
$$12\frac{4}{9}$$
$$-\ 7\frac{5}{6}$$

14.
$$1$$
$$-\ \frac{3}{7}$$

15.
$$30$$
$$-\ 15\frac{3}{7}$$

16.
$$34\frac{1}{20}$$
$$-\ 25\frac{8}{15}$$

17.
$$19\frac{1}{3}$$
$$-\ 14\frac{5}{6}$$

18.
$$12\frac{3}{20}$$
$$-\ 7\frac{7}{15}$$

19. $47\frac{3}{10} - 25\frac{5}{8}$ **20.** $8\frac{5}{12} - 5\frac{9}{10}$

Solve the following problems. After taking the test, see "Step-by-Step Solutions" for the answers (pages 239 to 241). And see "2.1 Fraction Terminology," "2.2 Multiplying Fractions," "2.3 Dividing Fractions," "2.4 Finding the Least Common Denominator (LCD)," "2.5 Adding Fractions," and "2.6 Subtracting Fractions," if the chapter test indicates you need additional practice.

Section 2.1

Change each improper fraction to a mixed number. Reduce if necessary.

1. $\dfrac{58}{5}$ 2. $\dfrac{23}{2}$ 3. $\dfrac{75}{6}$

Change each mixed number to an improper fraction.

4. $4\dfrac{6}{13}$ 5. $7\dfrac{3}{8}$

Section 2.2

Write answers in lowest form. Change improper fractions to mixed numbers.

6. $\dfrac{8}{9} \times \dfrac{54}{32}$ 7. $3\dfrac{4}{5} \times \dfrac{15}{4}$

8. $6 \times 5\dfrac{7}{8}$ 9. $\dfrac{3}{8} \times \dfrac{5}{6} \times \dfrac{16}{5}$

Section 2.3

10. $\dfrac{8}{15} \div \dfrac{4}{25}$ 11. $\dfrac{1}{2} \div 0$

12. $7\dfrac{7}{9} \div 3\dfrac{7}{21}$

Sections 2.4 and 2.5

13. $\dfrac{1}{5} + \dfrac{4}{5}$

14. $\begin{aligned} & 4\dfrac{1}{3} \\ +\ & 6\dfrac{3}{4} \\ \hline \end{aligned}$

15. $\dfrac{1}{3} + \dfrac{1}{8} + \dfrac{1}{9}$

16. $3\dfrac{3}{20} + 7\dfrac{7}{15} + 2\dfrac{1}{10}$

Sections 2.4 and 2.6

17. $\dfrac{5}{6} - \dfrac{3}{4}$

18. $\begin{aligned} & 7\dfrac{5}{6} \\ -\ & 4\dfrac{3}{14} \\ \hline \end{aligned}$

19. $\begin{aligned} & 5\dfrac{3}{8} \\ -\ & 2\dfrac{5}{8} \\ \hline \end{aligned}$

20. $\begin{aligned} & 16\dfrac{1}{8} \\ -\ & 13\dfrac{11}{12} \\ \hline \end{aligned}$

chapter 3

Decimal Numbers

3.0	**Pretest for Decimal Numbers**

Solve the following problems. After taking the test, see "Step-by-Step Solutions" for the answers (pages 242 to 243). Then, see "3.1 Place Value," "3.2 Rounding Decimal Numbers," "3.3 Adding and Subtracting Decimal Numbers," "3.4 Multiplying Decimal Numbers," "3.5 Dividing Decimal Numbers," "3.6 Converting Decimal Numbers and Fractions," and "3.7 Comparing Decimal Numbers and Fractions," for skill explanations.

Sections 3.1 and 3.2

1. Round 36.59 to the nearest tenth.

Section 3.3

2. 7.23 + 5.9614

3. 25.01 − 14.732

Section 3.4

4. 53.72 × 4.58

Section 3.5

Divide. Round the answer to the nearest tenth.

5. 376.42 ÷ 51.2

Section 3.6

6. Write 0.125 as a fraction in reduced form.

7. Change $\dfrac{4}{5}$ to a decimal.

Section 3.7

Arrange the decimal numbers from least to greatest.

8. 0.0119, 0.091, 0.0191, 0.01

Arrange the fractions from least to greatest.

9. $\dfrac{1}{5}, \dfrac{7}{15}, \dfrac{8}{25}$

Compare the fraction and decimal. Place <, =, or > in the blank.

10. $\dfrac{3}{25}$ _____ 0.14

3.1	**Place Value**

In this section, we will review:
- decimal numbers
- decimal points
- determining place value

Place Value System

We use the Hindu Arabic base 10-**place value** system, which has 10 different symbols to write numbers. The symbols, called **digits**, are—
0 1 2 3 4 5 6 7 8 9.

In this system, we understand that whole numbers, like 435 or 521, have a **decimal point** at the far right, the end—even though the decimal point is not visible. A **decimal number** contains a decimal point between the whole number and the decimal part. For example, 23.579 is a decimal number. We read a decimal point as *and*.

The following place value chart shows the names and values for each place on the chart. Note that the decimal point is in the middle and that it separates the whole numbers from the decimal part, sometimes called the **fractional part** of the number. (See Fig. 3.1.)

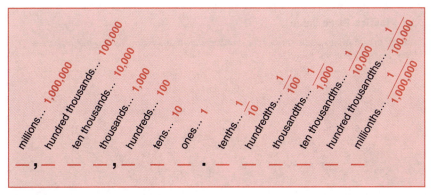

Figure 3.1. Understanding place value.

When reading or saying decimal numbers, use the place name of the number in the far-right position. For example, 0.8 is read as eight-tenths and 0.513 is read as five-hundred thirteen thousandths.

To determine the place value of a number, always start at the decimal point.

For Example:

If asked the place of each digit in 67.85, write the number below the place value names on the chart, being sure to place the decimal point correctly. (See Fig. 3.2.)

The answer: The 6 is in the tens' place, the 7 is in the ones' place, the 8 is in the tenths' place, and the 5 is in the hundredths' place.

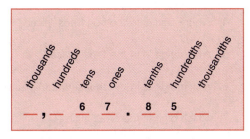

Figure 3.2. Placing the decimal point correctly.

3.1 Practice Place Value

Answer the following questions using the numbers shown and Figure 3.3. For the answers, see "Step-by-Step Solutions" (page 243).

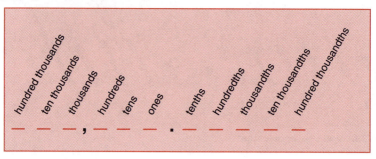

Figure 3.3. Place values.

4,328.576

1. Which digit is in the thousands' place?

2. Which digit is in the tenths' place?

3. Which digit is in the hundredths' place?

4. Which digit is in the hundreds' place?

5. Which digit is in the tens' place?

6. Which digit is in the thousandths' place?

7. Which digit is the ones' place?

853.92

8. Which digit is in the ones' place?

9. Which digit is in the hundreds' place?

10. Which digit is in the tenths' place?

11. Which digit is in the tens' place?

12. Which digit is in the hundredths' place?

32,804.1679

13. Which digit is in the thousands' place?

14. Which digit is in the tenths' place?

15. Which digit is in the ten thousandths' place?

16. Which digit is in the hundreds' place?

17. Which digit is in the ten thousands' place?

18. Which digit is in the tens' place?

19. Which digit is in the hundredths' place?

20. Which digit is in the ones' place?

3.2 **Rounding Decimal Numbers**

In this section, we will review:
- rounding whole and decimal numbers
- the circle and arrow rounding method

Rounding

Rounding is a kind of estimating that makes working with a number easier. We often use rounded number values when approximating money, time, and distance. For example, let's say you have $5.27. You might say, "I have about $5.00." This is rounding.

Numbers can be rounded to any place on a place value chart. (See Fig. 3.4.)

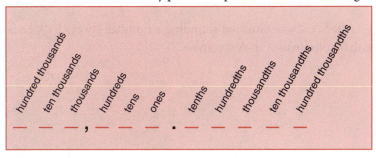

Figure 3.4. Rounding decimal numbers.

To round a whole or decimal number, follow these steps, using a circle ○ and an arrow ⇓.

1. Draw a circle around the digit in the place to which you are rounding.
2. Draw an arrow above the digit to its right.
3. Note that the circled digit either stays the same or increases by 1.
   - If the digit under the arrow is 4 or less (0, 1, 2, 3, 4), the circled digit stays the same.
   - If the digit under the arrow is 5 or greater (5, 6, 7, 8, 9), add 1 to the circled digit.

Example 1: Round 53,268 to the nearest thousand.

STEP 1. Circle the 3 in the thousands' place, and draw an arrow above the 2.

STEP 2. Do not change the 3 because the 2 is less than or equal to 4.

STEP 3. To complete the whole number, fill in the remaining places with zero(s) until you reach the decimal point.

The answer is 53,000.

$$5 \; ③, \overset{\Downarrow}{2} \; 6 \; 8$$

$$5 \; 3, \underline{0} \; \underline{0} \; \underline{0}$$

Example 2: Round 23.762 to the nearest tenth.

STEP 1. Circle the 7 in the tenths' place. Draw an arrow above the 6.

STEP 2. Increase the 7 to 8 because 6 is greater than or equal to 5.

The answer is 23.8.

$$2 \; 3. ⑦ \overset{\Downarrow}{6} \; 2$$

$$23.8$$

Tip: After you have finished rounding a number always look back to be sure that your answer makes sense.

3.2 Practice Rounding Decimal Numbers

Round the following numbers. For the answers, see "Step-by-Step Solutions" (page 244).
Mark appropriate numbers with a circle and an arrow.

1. Round 33.45 to the nearest tenth.

2. Round 74.561 to the nearest ten.

3. Round 234.357 to the nearest hundredth.

4. Round 25 to the nearest ten.

5. Round 36.758 to the nearest tenth.

6. Round 345.64 to the nearest tenth.

7. Round 34,785 to the nearest thousand.

8. Round 74.521 to the nearest one.

9. Round 345.856 to the nearest tenth.

10. Round 24.56 to the nearest one.

11. Round 456 to the nearest hundred.

12. Round 24.27614 to the nearest ten thousandth.

13. Round 76,476.23 to the nearest thousand.

14. Round 54 to the nearest ten.

15. Round 36.337 to the nearest hundredth.

16. Round 564 to the nearest hundred.

17. Round 1,362.2763 to the nearest thousandth.

18. Round 36.342 to the nearest one.

19. Round 24,776.25 to the nearest hundred.

20. Round 36,132 to the nearest thousand.

Adding and Subtracting Decimal Numbers

In this section, we will review:
- understanding the decimal point
- zero as a placeholder

Understanding the Decimal Point

All whole numbers have an understood decimal point at the far right, the end.

438 means 438.

5 means 5.

Zero as a Placeholder

Zero is used as a **placeholder** when adding and subtracting decimal numbers. Since all decimal numbers do not have the same number of decimal places, adding zero(s) to the end of the decimal part can make decimal numbers the same length. The zeros hold the place of the missing place value digits, keeping all digits in the correct column.

Adding

To add decimal numbers, follow these steps:

1. Line up the decimal points vertically (up and down) to guarantee that you are adding like place value units.
2. Fill missing decimal places with zeros as **placeholders** as shown. This step helps keep all numbers in the correct column.
3. Add as you do whole numbers. Be sure to bring down the decimal point.

Example 1:   4.7 + 3.25

STEP 1. Line up the decimal points vertically.

$$\begin{array}{r} 4.7 \\ + \ 3.25 \\ \hline \end{array}$$

STEP 2. Fill the missing decimal place in the 4.7 with a 0.

$$\begin{array}{r} 4.70 \\ + \ 3.25 \\ \hline \end{array}$$

STEP 3. Add the numbers. Bring down the decimal
point.

$$\begin{array}{r} 4.70 \\ + \ 3.25 \\ \hline 7.95 \end{array}$$

The answer is 7.95.

Example 2:   4 + 3.65 + 51.956

STEP 1. Line up the decimal points vertically.

$$\begin{array}{r} 4. \\ 3.65 \\ + \ 51.956 \end{array}$$

STEP 2. Fill the missing decimal places in the
4 and the 3.65 with 0s.

$$\begin{array}{r} 4.000 \\ 3.650 \\ + \ 51.956 \end{array}$$

STEP 3. Add the numbers. Bring down the decimal
point.

$$\begin{array}{r} 1 \ \ 1 \\ 4.000 \\ 3.650 \\ + \ 51.956 \\ \hline 59.606 \end{array}$$

The answer is 59.606.

Subtracting

To subtract decimal numbers, follow these steps:

1. Line up the decimal points vertically (up and down) to guarantee
   that you are subtracting like place-value units.
2. Fill missing decimal places with zeros as placeholders as shown.
   This step helps keep all numbers in the correct column.
3. Subtract as you would whole numbers. Bring down the decimal
   point.

Example 3: 5.637 − 4.32

STEP 1. Line up the decimal points vertically.

$$\begin{array}{r} 5.637 \\ -\ 4.32 \\ \hline \end{array}$$

STEP 2. Fill the missing decimal place in 4.32 with a 0.

$$\begin{array}{r} 5.637 \\ -\ 4.320 \\ \hline \end{array}$$

STEP 3. Subtract the numbers. Bring down the decimal point.

$$\begin{array}{r} 5.637 \\ -\ 4.320 \\ \hline 1.317 \end{array}$$

The answer is 1.317.

Example 4: 941.2 − 14.23

STEP 1. Line up the decimal points vertically.

$$\begin{array}{r} 941.2 \\ -\ 14.23 \\ \hline \end{array}$$

STEP 2. Fill the missing decimal place in 941.2 with a 0.

$$\begin{array}{r} 941.20 \\ -\ 14.23 \\ \hline \end{array}$$

STEP 3. Subtract the numbers, borrowing as needed. Bring down the decimal point.

$$\begin{array}{r} 3\ 10 \\ 0\ \ 11 \\ 1\ 10 \\ 9\cancel{4}\cancel{1}.\cancel{2}0 \\ -\ 1\ 4.23 \\ \hline 9\ 2\ 6.97 \end{array}$$

The answer is 926.97.

Example 5:   7 − 2.436

STEP 1. Line up the decimal points vertically.

$$
\begin{array}{r}
7.\;\;\; \\
-\,2.436
\end{array}
$$

STEP 2. Fill the missing decimal places in the
7 with 0s.

$$
\begin{array}{r}
7.000 \\
-\,2.436
\end{array}
$$

STEP 3. Subtract the numbers, borrowing as needed.
Bring down the decimal point.

$$
\begin{array}{r}
7.0\;0\;0 \\
-\,2.4\;3\;6 \\
\hline
4.5\;6\;4
\end{array}
$$

The answer is 4.564.

3.3 Practice Adding and Subtracting Decimal Numbers

Solve the following problems. For the answers, see "Step-by-Step Solutions" (pages 244 to 245).
Add.

1.   55.7
    + 23.2

2.   718.98
    + 496.69

3.   1.806
    + 4.856

Rewrite vertically; add.

4. 9.365 + 5.796

5. 79.061 + 5.72

6. 813.7 + 629.86

7. 1.86 + 23.2

8. 26.905 + 7,643.457

9. 6.543 + 12.61 + 304.8

10. 18.297 + 7.6 + 199.83

Subtract.

11.
```
  7 6
- 4.8
```

12.
```
  82.3
- 43.94
```

13.
```
  185.47
-  67.5
```

Rewrite vertically; subtract.

14. 243.98 − 84.256

15. 4,986.25 − 3,615.24

16. 12 − 1.263

17. 1.5 − 0.03752

18. 25.754 − 25.752

19. 17.54 − 2.0432

20. 100.232 − 0.4

| 3.4 | **Multiplying Decimal Numbers** |

In this section, we will review:
- calculating the number of decimal places in a product
- trailing zeros
- zero preceding a decimal point

Knowing the Process

To multiply with decimal numbers, follow these steps:

1. Write the problem vertically as if you were working with whole numbers, writing the longest number (the one with the most digits) on the top. Align the second number with the far right side of the top number.
2. Multiply as you do whole numbers.
3. Determine the number of decimal places in the answer by adding the number of decimal places in both factors. Start at the far right of the product and draw small arrows to the left the total number of decimal places that the answer needs.
4. Write the answer in best mathematical form.

Trailing Zeros

In the decimal part of a number, zeros to the right of the last nonzero digit (1, 2, 3, 4, 5, 6, 7, 8, or 9) are called **trailing zeros**. For example, 65.2300 has two trailing zeros. The 0 in the thousandths' place and the 0 in the ten-thousandths' place have no value. To write an answer like 65.2300 in best mathematical form, drop the trailing zeros. Write the answer as 65.23.

Zero Preceding a Decimal Point

For answers with only a decimal part, place a zero to the left of the decimal point so the answer is in best mathematical form. It is easy to miss seeing a decimal point. The zero makes the decimal point stand out. In medication dosages, clear communication is essential. If a decimal point is not noticed, a dosage error could occur. For example, reading .5 mL as 5 mL results in a tenfold dosage error. Writing 0.5 mL helps to avoid human error.

Example 1: 3.46×0.5

STEP 1. Write the problem vertically.

$$
\begin{array}{r}
3.46 \\
\times\, 0.5 \\
\end{array}
$$

STEP 2. Multiply as you do whole numbers.

$$
\begin{array}{r}
^{2\ 3} \\
3.46 \\
\times\, 0.5 \\
\hline
1730 \\
\end{array}
$$

STEP 3. Add the number of decimal places in the two factors: The 3.46 has two decimal places, and 0.5 has one decimal place, so the total is three decimal places. The answer will have three decimal places.

$$\begin{array}{r} \overset{2\ 3}{3.46} \\ \times\ 0.5 \\ \hline 1.730 \end{array}$$

STEP 4. Insert the decimal point three places to the left as shown with the arrows.

STEP 5. Drop the trailing 0 and write the answer in best mathematical form.

$$1.730 = 1.73$$

The answer is 1.73.

Example 2: $\begin{array}{r} 5.41 \\ \times\ 0.12 \\ \hline \end{array}$

STEP 1. Multiply as you do whole numbers.

$$\begin{array}{r} 5.41 \\ \times\ 0.12 \\ \hline 1082 \\ 541 \\ \hline 6492 \end{array}$$

STEP 2. Count the decimal places in the two factors: Each has two decimal places, so the total is four decimal places.

$$\begin{array}{r} 5.41 \\ \times\ 0.12 \\ \hline 1082 \\ 541 \\ \hline .6492 \end{array}$$

STEP 3. Insert the decimal point four places to the left as shown with the arrows.

STEP 4. Place a 0 to the left of the decimal point.

$$0.6492$$

The answer is 0.6492.

After multiplying two decimal numbers, if the product does not have enough decimal places, then move to the left drawing arrows until you reach the desired decimal point placement. Next write zeros in the blank places. Also, remember to write a zero to the left of the decimal point.

Example 3:   0.004
               × 0.02

STEP 1. Multiply as you do whole numbers.

$$\begin{array}{r} \mathbf{0.004} \\ \times\ \mathbf{0.02} \\ \hline \mathbf{8} \end{array}$$

STEP 2. Count the decimal places in the two factors: The 0.004 has three decimal places, and the 0.02 has two decimal places, so the total is five decimal places.

STEP 3. Insert the decimal point five places to left as shown with the arrows. Fill in four zeros to the left of the 8 to make five decimal places.

$$\begin{array}{r} \mathbf{0.004} \\ \times\ \mathbf{0.02} \\ \hline \mathbf{.00008} \end{array}$$

STEP 4. Place a 0 to the left of the decimal point.

0.00008

The answer is 0.00008.

3.4 Practice Multiplying Decimal Numbers

Solve the following problems. For the answers, see "Step-by-Step Solutions" (pages 245 to 246).
Multiply.

1. 0.6 × 0.9	2. 0.13 × 0.5	3. 0.028 × 0.89	4. 0.0437 × 0.48
5. 6.234 × 2.25	6. 81.26 × 4.89	7. 924.3 × 96.4	8. 9.6501 × 129.8
9. 19.07 × 0.05	10. 5,167 × 0.19	11. 2.163 × 0.008	12. 0.6718 × 50.04

Rewrite in vertical form, then multiply.

13. 126 × 3.5

14. 5,060 × 9.57

15. $7{,}090 \times 1.74$ **16.** 0.06×0.07

17. 70.92×2.05 **18.** 8.703×8.08

19. $0.001 \times 6{,}523.7$ **20.** 0.07×0.0056

<table>
<tr><td>3.5</td><td>

Dividing Decimal Numbers

</td></tr>
</table>

In this section, we will review:
* changing a decimal number to a whole number
* rounding decimal quotients

The Process

To divide by decimal numbers, first recall division terminology:

$$\text{divisor}\,\overline{)\,\text{dividend}}^{\text{quotient}}$$

. Then follow these steps:

1. Change the decimal number in the divisor to a whole number because you can divide by whole numbers only. (In other words, you cannot divide by a decimal number.) To make the change, move the decimal point to the right until the divisor becomes a whole number. Actually, you are multiplying by powers of 10 as you move the decimal point to the right.

   For example, if the divisor is 64.3 move the decimal point one place to the right (64.3.). You are actually multiplying by 10 to make the whole number 643. And for a divisor of 0.42 move the decimal point two places to the right (0.42.) or multiply by 100 to make the whole number 42.

2. Whatever you do to the divisor, you have to do to the dividend. So, move the decimal point in the dividend to the right as well. Move the same number of decimal places as you did in the divisor.

$$4.23.\overline{)64.27.}$$

3. Add zeros if needed to fill to the new placement of the decimal point. $23.456\overline{)69.2}$ should be rewritten as $23.456.\overline{)69.200.}$

4. Place the decimal point in the quotient directly above the new decimal point in the dividend.

5. Divide as you do whole numbers. Keep dividing until you reach the decimal point as shown in Example 1. If needed, after all division is completed, place zeros in the answer (quotient) to reach the decimal point.

Example 1: 45 ÷ 0.03

STEP 1. Write the problem so that the dividend is under the division symbol and the divisor is to the left of the symbol.

$$0.03\overline{)45}$$

STEP 2. Change the decimal number in the divisor to a whole number.

$$0.03.\overline{)45}$$

STEP 3. Move the decimal point in the dividend to the right.

$$0.03.\overline{)45..}$$

STEP 4. Add 0s to the dividend.

$$0.03.\overline{)4500.}$$

STEP 5. Place the decimal point in the quotient directly above the new decimal point in the dividend.

$$0.03.\overline{)4500.}$$

STEP 6. Divide as you do whole numbers, placing the decimal point in the quotient above the new decimal point in the dividend.

$$
\begin{array}{r}
1{,}500. \\
0.03.\overline{)4500.} \\
\underline{-3} \\
15 \\
\underline{-15} \\
000
\end{array}
$$

The answer is 1,500.

Rounding to Certain Places

Example 1 works out evenly. However, in problems that do not work out evenly, the instructions will indicate if you should round the quotient. (For basic rounding rules, see page 61.)

If the instructions say:

- round the quotient to the nearest whole number, divide until you have a number in the tenths' place, then round to the nearest whole number.
- round the quotient to the nearest tenth, divide until you have a number in the hundredths' place, then round to the nearest tenth.
- round the quotient to the nearest hundredth, divide until you have a number in the thousandths' place, then round to the nearest hundredth.
- round the quotient to the nearest thousandth, divide until you have a number in the ten thousandths' place, then round to the nearest thousandth.

Example 2: Round the quotient to the nearest tenth.

$$32.4974 \div 4.8$$

STEP 1. Write the problem so that the dividend is under the division symbol and the divisor is to the left of the symbol.

$$4.8 \overline{)32.4974}$$

STEP 2. Change the decimal number in the divisor to a whole number.

$$4.8. \overline{)32.4974}$$

STEP 3. Move the decimal point in the dividend to the right.

$$4.8. \overline{)32.4.974}$$

STEP 4. Place the decimal point in the quotient directly above the new decimal point in the dividend.

$$4.8. \overline{)32.4.974}$$

STEP 5. Divide as you do whole numbers. Continue dividing until you reach the hundredths' place since the instructions are to round to the nearest tenth.

$$
\begin{array}{r}
6.77 \\
4.8.)\overline{32.4.974} \\
-288 \\
\hline
369 \\
-336 \\
\hline
337 \\
-336 \\
\hline
1
\end{array}
$$

STEP 6. Round 6.77 to the nearest tenth.

$6.\textcircled{7}7 = 6.8$

The answer is 6.8.

Example 3: Round the quotient to the nearest hundredth.
47.4 ÷ 23.2

STEP 1. Write the problem so the dividend is under the division symbol and the divisor is to the left of the symbol.

$23.2)\overline{47.4}$

STEP 2. Change the decimal number in the divisor to a whole number.

$23.2.)\overline{47.4}$

STEP 3. Move the decimal point in the dividend to the right.

$23.2.)\overline{47.4.}$

STEP 4. Place the decimal point in the quotient directly above the new decimal point in the dividend.

$23.2.)\overline{47.4.}$

STEP 5. Add three 0s as shown so that you can round the answer to the nearest hundredth.

$23.2.)\overline{47.4.000}$

STEP 6. Divide as you do whole numbers.
Continue dividing until you reach the
thousandths' place.

$$
\begin{array}{r}
2.043 \\
23.2.\overline{\smash{)}47.4.000} \\
-464 \\
\hline
1000 \\
-928 \\
\hline
720 \\
-696 \\
\hline
24
\end{array}
$$

STEP 7. Round 2.043 to the nearest hundredth. 2.0④3 = 2.04

The answer is 2.04.

3.5 Practice Dividing Decimal Numbers

Solve the following problems. For the answers, see "Step-by-Step Solutions" (pages 247 to 249).
Divide until the remainder is zero.

1. $4\overline{)0.044}$ 2. $5\overline{)0.0129}$ 3. $64\overline{)3.616}$ 4. $0.5\overline{)32.15}$

5. $12.2\overline{)9.76}$ 6. $0.85\overline{)41.905}$ 7. $1.87\overline{)170.6562}$ 8. $0.69\overline{)8.44974}$

9. $0.8113 \div 0.07$ 10. $40.3 \div 0.31$ 11. $95.20 \div 0.28$ 12. $75.6 \div 3.6$

Round each quotient to the nearest tenth.

13. $0.023\overline{)65.226}$ 14. $7.05\overline{)0.4977}$ 15. $1.33\overline{)75}$

Round each quotient to the nearest hundredth.

16. $26\overline{)5.729}$ 17. $3.181\overline{)6}$ 18. $1.23\overline{)14.91129}$

Round each quotient to the nearest thousandth.

19. $2.57\overline{)0.4961}$ **20.** $0.23\overline{)45.576}$

Converting Decimal Numbers and Fractions

In this section, we will review:
- changing a decimal number to a fraction
- changing a fraction to a decimal number
- repeating decimal numbers

Changing a Decimal Number to a Fraction

To change a decimal number to a fraction recall how decimal numbers are read. (See Fig. 3.5 and Section 3.1, "Place Value")

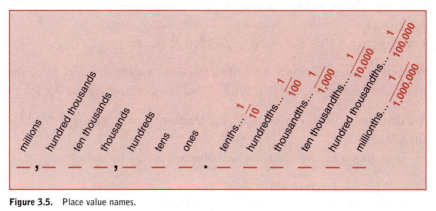

Figure 3.5. Place value names.

To write a decimal number in fraction form, follow the process shown in Table 3.1.

Table 3.1: From Decimal Number to Fraction		
Decimal number	**Read as …**	**Fraction or reduced fraction form**
0.3	3 tenths	$\dfrac{3}{10}$
0.45	45 hundredths	$\dfrac{45}{100} = \dfrac{9}{20}$
16.5	16 and 5 tenths	$16\dfrac{5}{10} = 16\dfrac{1}{2}$
324.125	324 and 125 thousandths	$324\dfrac{125}{1000} = 324\dfrac{1}{8}$

As you can see from the table above, the fraction form is a mixed number when a decimal number consists of a whole number part and a fraction part. Always reduce fractions for the final answer.

Changing a Fraction to a Decimal Number

A fraction means division. To write a fraction to show division, place the numerator under the division symbol and the denominator to the left of

the division symbol. For example, the fraction $\dfrac{1}{5}$ is written $5\overline{)1}$ to show division.

To change a fraction to a decimal number, follow these steps:

1. Write the fraction as division.
2. Add a decimal point and zero(s) to the dividend as needed.
3. Divide.

Example 1: Write $\dfrac{1}{4}$ as a decimal number.

STEP 1. The fraction $\dfrac{1}{4}$ means 1 divided by 4.

$$4\overline{)1}$$

STEP 2. Add a decimal point and zeros to begin dividing.

$$4\overline{)1.00}$$

STEP 3. Divide.

$$
\begin{array}{r}
0.25 \\
4\overline{)1.00} \\
-8 \\
\hline
20 \\
-20 \\
\hline
0
\end{array}
$$

The answer is $\frac{1}{4} = 0.25$.

Example 2: Write $\frac{2}{3}$ as a decimal number.

STEP 1. The fraction $\frac{2}{3}$ means 2 divided by 3.

$$3\overline{)2}$$

STEP 2. Add a decimal point and zeros to begin dividing.

$$3\overline{)2.00}$$

STEP 3. Divide.

$$
\begin{array}{r}
0.66 \\
3\overline{)2.00} \\
-18 \\
\hline
20 \\
-18 \\
\hline
2
\end{array}
$$

STEP 4. This division problem does not end since you keep getting a remainder of 2.

The answer written in best mathematical form is $0.\overline{6}$.

Repeating Decimal Numbers

When the digits in the decimal part of a decimal number repeat, as in the fraction $\frac{2}{3}$, the decimal number is called a **repeating decimal number**.

New Notation

A bar, like ‾, is placed over repeating digits to indicate a repeating pattern in the decimal part of a decimal number.

Other fractions that result in repeating decimals when divided are as shown.

$$\frac{1}{6} = 0.1666 \ldots = 0.1\overline{6}$$

$$\frac{1}{11} = 0.0909 \ldots = 0.\overline{09}$$

$$\frac{1}{7} = 0.142857142857 \ldots = 0.\overline{142857}$$

New Notation

Three dots placed ... mean *and so forth* in mathematical notation.

3.6 Practice Converting Decimal Numbers and Fractions

Solve the following problems. For the answers, see "Step-by-Step Solutions" (pages 249 to 250).
Change each decimal number to a fraction or a mixed number. Reduce if necessary.

1. 0.25

2. 17.7

3. 0.375

4. 0.2

5. 865.75

6. 0.625

7. 34.5

8. 0.35

9. 5.09

10. 0.075

Change the following fractions to a decimal number.

11. $\dfrac{4}{5}$

12. $\dfrac{1}{3}$

---

13. $\dfrac{5}{8}$

14. $\dfrac{1}{5}$

15. $\dfrac{1}{4}$

16. $\dfrac{3}{4}$

17. $\dfrac{7}{20}$

18. $\dfrac{9}{25}$

19. $\dfrac{2}{5}$

20. $\dfrac{3}{8}$

3.7   **Comparing Decimal Numbers and Fractions**

In this section, we will review:
- trailing zeros
- least common denominator

Trailing Zeros

Adding trailing zeros to the decimal part of a decimal number does not change the value of the number. The decimal numbers 25.7, 25.70, and 25.700 all have the same value.

Comparing Decimal Numbers

To compare decimal numbers, determine which decimal number has the most decimal places. Add trailing zeros to each of the other decimal numbers so they contain an equal number of decimal places. Then, compare the numbers. Write the answer with the original decimal numbers given in the problem.

Example 1: Order the decimal numbers 1.8, 1.06, and 1.732 from least to greatest.

STEP 1. Determine the decimal number with the largest number of decimal places. The decimal number 1.732 has three decimal places.

STEP 2. Write the decimal numbers with three decimal places by adding trailing zeros, if needed.

1.800
1.060
1.732

STEP 3. Arrange the numbers from least to greatest.

1.060
1.732
1.800

STEP 4. Remove the trailing zeros. Write the original decimal numbers from least to greatest.

1.06
1.732
1.8

The answer is 1.06, 1.732, 1.8.

Comparing Fractions

Before comparing fractions, find their least common denominator. Replace each fraction with its equivalent fraction containing the least common denominator. Then compare the numerators. Write the answer with the original fractions in the problem.

Example 2: Order from least to greatest $\dfrac{1}{2}, \dfrac{3}{4}, \dfrac{5}{8}$

STEP 1. Find the least common denominator of 2, 4, and 8.

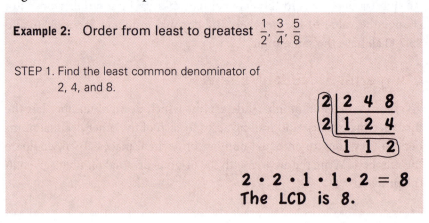

$$2 \cdot 2 \cdot 1 \cdot 1 \cdot 2 = 8$$
The LCD is 8.

STEP 2. Write equivalent fractions with a denominator of 8.

$$\frac{1}{2} = \frac{4}{8}$$

$$\frac{3}{4} = \frac{6}{8}$$

$$\frac{5}{8} = \frac{5}{8}$$

STEP 3. Write the fractions with their numerators in order from least to greatest.

$$\frac{4}{8}, \frac{5}{8}, \frac{6}{8}$$

STEP 4. Write the corresponding fractions from the original problem in order from least to greatest.

$$\frac{1}{2}, \frac{5}{8}, \frac{3}{4}$$

The answer is $\frac{1}{2}, \frac{5}{8}, \frac{3}{4}$.

Comparing a Fraction and a Decimal Number

To compare a fraction and a decimal number, first convert the fraction to a decimal number by performing division. Add trailing zeros if needed. Then compare the two decimal numbers using a less than (<) or greater than (>) symbol.

New Notation

The < symbol means less than, and the > symbol means greater than.

Example 3: Compare $\frac{3}{4}$ and 0.627

STEP 1. Convert $\frac{3}{4}$ to a decimal number by performing division.

$$4\overline{)3.00} = 0.75$$

STEP 2. Write the two decimal numbers with the same number of decimal places adding trailing zeros if needed.

0.750
0.627

STEP 3. Insert the correct symbol to make a true statement.

STEP 4. Write the corresponding fraction for the decimal number 0.750.

$$0.750 > 0.627$$

$$\frac{3}{4} > 0.627$$

The answer is $\frac{3}{4} > 0.627$.

3.7 Practice Comparing Decimal Numbers and Fractions

Solve the following problems. For the answers, see "Step-by-Step Solutions" (pages 250 to 253).

Arrange the decimal numbers from least to greatest.

1. 0.263, 0.2632, 0.26, 0.2

2. 0.473, 0.472, 0.4, 0.4732

3. 0.074, 0.07421, 0.0744, 0.0724

4. 0.26262, 0.6262, 0.62, 0.262

5. 0.24, 0.21, 0.401, 0.241

6. 0.0426, 0.4, 0.0461, 0.06

Arrange the fractions from least to greatest.

7. $\frac{2}{3}, \frac{1}{2}, \frac{5}{6}$ 8. $\frac{5}{24}, \frac{11}{15}, \frac{7}{30}$ 9. $\frac{7}{12}, \frac{1}{21}, \frac{2}{3}$ 10. $\frac{5}{16}, \frac{11}{18}, \frac{1}{24}$

11. $\frac{7}{15}, \frac{11}{12}, \frac{7}{8}$ 12. $\frac{1}{8}, \frac{3}{4}, \frac{9}{16}$ 13. $\frac{2}{5}, \frac{1}{4}, \frac{7}{15}$

Compare these fractions and decimals. Place <, =, or > in the blank.

14. 0.627 ___ $\frac{5}{8}$ 15. 0.3 ___ $\frac{1}{4}$ 16. $\frac{7}{20}$ ___ 0.36

17. $\frac{19}{40}$ ___ 0.47   18. $\frac{3}{4}$ ___ 0.75   19. $\frac{3}{5}$ ___ 0.56

20. 0.28 ___ $\frac{7}{25}$

Solve the following problems. After taking the test, see "Step-by-Step Solutions" for the answers (pages 254 to 255). And see "3.1 Place Value," "3.2 Rounding Decimals," "3.3 Adding and Subtracting Decimals," "3.4 Multiplying Decimals," "3.5 Dividing Decimals," "3.6 Converting Decimal Numbers and Fractions," and "3.7 Comparing Decimal Numbers and Fractions" if the chapter test indicates you need additional practice.

Section 3.1

1. Which digit is in the thousandths' place? 0.2963

2. Which digit is in the tens' place? 5,642.3

Sections 3.1 and 3.2

3. Round 3.451 to the nearest hundredth.

4. Round 57.85 to the nearest tenth.

Section 3.3

5. 4.56 + 2.3

6. 1.942 + 0.23 + 67.897

7. 567.259 − 43.8715

8. 73 − 7.596

Section 3.4

9.   67.5
    × 0.84

10. 0.07 × 0.0063

Section 3.5

11. $7.29\overline{)47.385}$

12. Divide. Round to the nearest tenth. $1.45\overline{)75}$

Section 3.6

13. Write 0.6 in fraction form.

14. Change $\dfrac{5}{8}$ to a decimal number.

Section 3.7

Arrange the decimal numbers from least to greatest.

15. 0.0893, 0.9, 0.0839, 0.89

16. 1.525, 1.51, 1.526, 1.54

Arrange the fractions from least to greatest.

17. $\dfrac{5}{9}, \dfrac{3}{4}, \dfrac{11}{18}$

18. $\dfrac{3}{7}, \dfrac{4}{21}, \dfrac{16}{35}$

Compare these fractions and decimals. Place <, =, or > in the blank.

19. 0.23 ___ $\dfrac{11}{50}$

20. 0.69 ___ $\dfrac{7}{10}$

chapter 4

Percents, Ratios, and Proportions

4.0   Pretest for Percents, Ratios, and Proportions

Solve the following problems. After taking the test, see "Step-by-Step Solutions" for the answers (pages 256 to 257). Then, see "4.1 Ratios and Proportions," "4.2 The Percent Proportion," "4.3 Fractions, Ratios, and Percents," and "4.4 Working with Percents and Decimal Numbers," for skill explanations.

Section 4.1

Solve the proportion for x.

1. $\dfrac{8}{3} = \dfrac{x}{15}$

Section 4.2

Use the percent proportion to solve for x.

2. x is 5% of 50.

3. 40 is 20% of x.

4. $\dfrac{1}{2}$ is what percent of $\dfrac{3}{4}$?

5. Write 62.5% as a fraction in reduced form.

6. Write $\frac{4}{5}$ as a percent.

7. Write the ratio 8:40 as a percent.

Section 4.4

8. Change 500% to a decimal number.

9. Change 7.98 to a percent.

10. $\frac{8.6}{40\%}$

4.1

Ratios and Proportions

In this section, we will review:
- cross multiplying
- cross products
- finding the value of x in a proportion

Ratios and Proportions

A **ratio** is a comparison of two numbers. A ratio can be written in several forms.

$$2 \text{ to } 3 \qquad 2:3 \qquad \frac{2}{3}$$

Before using a ratio in a proportion problem, write it in fraction form.

$$3:4 \qquad \frac{3}{4} \qquad 7 \text{ to } 8 \qquad \frac{7}{8}$$

Proportion Terminology

A **proportion** is a true statement in which two ratios are equal.

For example, $\frac{5}{6} = \frac{25}{30}$ is a proportion.

Each term in a proportion is referred to as either a mean or extreme depending on its location in the proportion: $\frac{extreme}{mean} = \frac{mean}{extreme}$. For example, in the proportion $\frac{5}{6} = \frac{25}{30}$, 5 and 30 are the extremes and 6 and 25 are the means.

Cross Multiplying

The method of multiplying in a proportion is called cross multiplying. Cross multiplying is shown in a proportion using an $\times$.

When the means and extremes in a proportion are multiplied, they result in **cross products.** The cross products in a proportion are equal. For example, $5 \cdot 30 = 150$ and $6 \cdot 25 = 150$.

Tip: Be careful not to confuse cross canceling with cross multiplying. Cross canceling is used when multiplying fractions; cross multiplying is used when multiplying means and extremes in proportions.

Proving that a Proportion is True

A proportion is true if the cross products are equal.

These steps prove that a proportion is true.

$$\frac{5}{6} \times \frac{25}{30}$$

$$5 \cdot 30 = 25 \cdot 6$$
$$150 = 150$$

If the cross products are not equal after cross multiplying, the proportion is not true.

Conditional Proportion

When one part of a proportion is a **variable** (a letter such as x), the proportion is a **conditional proportion**. It is not true or false, but there is a value of x that will make it true. You can place the x **(unknown)** in any position in the proportion. And you can write the same proportion in four ways by changing the placement of the x.

$$\frac{x}{2} = \frac{5}{10} \qquad \frac{1}{x} = \frac{5}{10} \qquad \frac{1}{2} = \frac{x}{10} \qquad \frac{1}{2} = \frac{5}{x}$$

Steps for Solving a Proportion

Proportions may contain many kinds of numbers including whole numbers, fractions, decimal numbers, and negative numbers. Regardless of the types of numbers in a proportion, you can solve all proportions by following the same basic steps. As you can see in the examples, you can combine some of the steps when actually solving the problem.

1. Cross multiply the means or extremes, so that the cross multiplication containing x is on the left side of the equation. Then set it equal to the remaining cross multiplication.
2. Perform the multiplication to find the cross products.
3. Divide both sides by the number in front of the x.
4. Simplify the answer. The answer is the value of x that makes the proportion true.

Example 1: $\dfrac{5}{20} = \dfrac{1}{x}$

STEP 1. Cross multiply the extremes so the variable, x, is on the left side of the equation. Set it equal to the remaining cross multiplication.

$$5 \cdot x = 1 \cdot 20$$

STEP 2. Perform the multiplication to find the cross products.

$$5x = 20$$

STEP 3. Divide both sides by the number in front of the x.

$$\dfrac{\cancel{5}^{1}x}{\cancel{5}_{1}} = \dfrac{\cancel{20}^{4}}{\cancel{5}_{1}}$$

STEP 4. Simplify the answer.

$$1x = 4$$
$$x = 4$$

The answer is x = 4.

Tip: In best mathematical form, 1x is written as x. It is understood that there is a 1 in front of any variable (letter) like x. For example, y means 1y and g means 1g.

Example 2: $\dfrac{3}{8} = \dfrac{x}{21}$

STEP 1. Cross multiply the means so the variable, x, is on the left side of the equation. Set it equal to the remaining cross multiplication.

$$8 \cdot x = 3 \cdot 21$$

STEP 2. Perform the multiplication to find the cross products.

$$8x = 63$$

STEP 3. Divide both sides by the number in front of the x.

$$\frac{\overset{1}{\cancel{8}}x}{\underset{1}{\cancel{8}}} = \frac{63}{8}$$

STEP 4. Simplify the answer by changing the improper fraction to a mixed number.

$$x = \frac{63}{8}$$

$$x = 7\frac{7}{8}$$

The answer is $7\frac{7}{8}$.

Example 3: $\frac{x}{4} = \frac{3}{2}$

STEP 1. Cross multiply the extremes so the variable, x, is on the left side of the equation. Set it equal to the remaining cross multiplication.

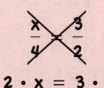

$$2 \cdot x = 3 \cdot 4$$

STEP 2. Perform the multiplication to find the cross products.

$$2x = 12$$

STEP 3. Divide both sides by the number in front of the x.

$$\frac{\overset{1}{\cancel{2}}x}{\underset{1}{\cancel{2}}} = \frac{\overset{6}{\cancel{12}}}{\underset{1}{\cancel{2}}}$$

STEP 4. Simplify the answer.

$$x = 6$$

The answer is 6.

4.1 Practice Ratios and Proportions

Solve the following proportions. For the answers, see "Step-by-Step Solutions" (pages 257 to 258). Solve each proportion for the unknown variable.

1. $\dfrac{2}{7} = \dfrac{x}{42}$

2. $\dfrac{3}{2} = \dfrac{12}{y}$

3. $\dfrac{k}{8} = \dfrac{8}{9}$

4. $\dfrac{6}{z} = \dfrac{3}{5}$

5. $\dfrac{2}{5} = \dfrac{3}{w}$

6. $\dfrac{x}{3} = \dfrac{3}{2}$

7. $\dfrac{3}{5} = \dfrac{15}{n}$

8. $\dfrac{1}{4} = \dfrac{x}{44}$

9. $\dfrac{n}{5} = \dfrac{6}{15}$

10. $\dfrac{3}{4} = \dfrac{16}{n}$

11. $\dfrac{n}{9} = \dfrac{1}{3}$

12. $\dfrac{3}{x} = \dfrac{15}{25}$

13. $\dfrac{3}{24} = \dfrac{k}{8}$

14. $\dfrac{n}{32} = \dfrac{15}{16}$

15. $\dfrac{7}{10} = \dfrac{20}{x}$

16. $\dfrac{x}{9} = \dfrac{25}{100}$

17. $\dfrac{9}{n} = \dfrac{3}{20}$

18. $\dfrac{n}{10} = \dfrac{2}{5}$

19. $\dfrac{16}{n} = \dfrac{7}{25}$

20. $\dfrac{3}{n} = \dfrac{7}{25}$

The Percent Proportion

In this section, we will review:
- the meaning of percent
- using the percent proportion to find x

Percent means "parts of 100." This can be represented by the fraction $\frac{x}{100}$.

For example, on a test if you score 89 out of 100 points, you have scored $\frac{89}{100}$ or 89%.

In some types of applied problems you encounter in nursing, you will need to know how to work with percents.

The Percent Proportion

The **percent proportion** is written $\frac{is}{of} = \frac{percent}{100}$. These are the meanings of the terms:

The word *is* represents part of a number.

The word *of* represents the whole number.

The word *percent* represents the percent.

In the following percent problems, the wording tells you where to place the information in the percent proportion. These are the basic steps to solve a percent problem. However, if the problem has fractions or decimal numbers, additional steps may be needed.

1. Substitute the given information into the percent proportion.
2. Cross multiply and place the variable on the left side of the equation.
3. Divide both sides by the number to the left of the x.
4. Simplify the answer. Be sure to write the answer as a percent, if needed.

Example 1: 6 is what % of 24?

STEP 1. Substitute the given information into the percent proportion.
6 *is* - substitute 6 for *is*
what % - substitute x for *percent*
of 24 - substitute 24 for *of*.
Fill in *100*.

$$\frac{6\,(is)}{(of)\,24} = \frac{x\,(percent)}{100}$$

STEP 2. Cross multiply and place the variable on the left side of the equation.

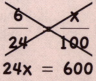

$$24x = 600$$

STEP 3. Divide both sides by the number to the left of the x.

$$\frac{\overset{1}{\cancel{24}}x}{\underset{1}{\cancel{24}}} = \frac{600}{24} \qquad 24\overline{)600}^{\,25}$$

STEP 4. Simplify the answer. Write the answer as a percent, if needed.

$$x = 25\%$$

The answer is 25%.

Example 2: 80 is 20% of x.

STEP 1. Substitute the given information into the percent proportion.
80 is - substitute 80 for *is*
20% - substitute 20 for *percent*
of x - substitute x for *of*
Fill in *100*.

$$\frac{80\,(is)}{(of)\,x} = \frac{20\,(percent)}{100}$$

STEP 2. Cross multiply. Place the variable on the left side of the equation.

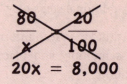

$$20x = 8,000$$

STEP 3. Divide both sides by the number to the left of the x.

$$\frac{\overset{1}{\cancel{20}}x}{\underset{1}{\cancel{20}}} = \frac{8,000}{20}$$

$$20\overline{)8,000}^{\,400}$$

STEP 4. Simplify the answer. Write the answer as a percent, if needed.

$$x = 400$$

The answer is 400.

Example 3: 24% of 375 = what?

STEP 1. Substitute the given information into the percent proportion.
24% - substitute 24 for *percent*
of 375 - substitute 375 for *of*
= means is - substitute x for *is*
Fill in *100*.

$$\frac{x\,(is)}{(of)\,375} = \frac{24\,(percent)}{100}$$

STEP 2. Cross multiply and place the variable on the left side of the equation.

$$\frac{x}{375} \,\,\diagdown\!\!\!\!\diagup\,\, \frac{24}{100}$$

$$100x = 9,000$$

STEP 3. Divide both sides by the number to the left of the x.

$$\frac{\cancel{100}^1\,x}{\cancel{100}_1} = \frac{9,000}{100}$$

$$100\overline{)9,000} \quad \overset{90}{}$$

STEP 4. Simplify the answer.

$$x = 90$$

The answer is 90.

Example 4: $\frac{3}{8}$ is ?% of $\frac{5}{4}$.

STEP 1. Substitute the given information into the percent proportion.
$\frac{3}{8}$ *is* – substitute $\frac{3}{8}$ for *is*.

?% means what percent. Substitute x for *percent*.

of $\frac{5}{4}$ – substitute $\frac{5}{4}$ for *of*.

Fill in *100*.

$$\frac{\frac{3}{8}\,(is)}{(of)\,\frac{5}{4}} = \frac{x\,(?\%)}{100}$$

STEP 2. Cross multiply and place the variable
on the left side of the equation.

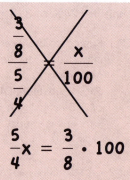

$$\frac{5}{4}x = \frac{3}{8} \cdot 100$$

STEP 3. Write the whole number 100 in fraction
form.

$$\frac{5}{4}x = \frac{3}{8} \cdot \frac{100}{1}$$

STEP 4. To obtain 1x, multiply both sides
by $\frac{4}{5}$, the reciprocal of $\frac{5}{4}$.

$$\frac{4}{5} \cdot \frac{5}{4}x = \frac{300}{8} \cdot \frac{4}{5}$$

STEP 5. Cross cancel, then
multiply

$$\frac{\overset{1}{\cancel{4}}}{\underset{1}{\cancel{5}}} \cdot \frac{\overset{1}{\cancel{5}}}{\underset{1}{\cancel{4}}}x = \frac{\overset{30}{\cancel{\overset{60}{\cancel{300}}}}}{\underset{1}{\cancel{\underset{2}{\cancel{8}}}}} \cdot \frac{\overset{1}{\cancel{4}}}{\underset{1}{\cancel{5}}}$$

STEP 6. Simplify the answer. Write the
answer as a percent, if needed.
x = 30%.

$$x = 30\%$$

The answer is 30%.

To solve a problem that contains both a fraction and a decimal number, rewrite one of the terms so the problem has either two fractions or two decimal numbers.

Example 5: $2\frac{1}{2}$% of what is 0.16?

STEP 1. Write 0.16 as a fraction.

$$0.16 = \frac{16}{100} = \frac{4}{25}$$

STEP 2. Rewrite the problem.

$$2\frac{1}{2}\% \text{ of what is } \frac{4}{25}?$$

STEP 3. Substitute the given information into the percent proportion.

$$\frac{\frac{4}{25}}{x} = \frac{2\frac{1}{2}}{100}$$

STEP 4. Change the mixed number to an improper fraction.

$$\frac{\frac{4}{25}}{x} \diagup\!\!\!\!\diagdown \frac{\frac{5}{2}}{100}$$

STEP 5. Cross multiply and place the variable on the left side of the equation.

$$\frac{5}{2}x = \frac{4}{25} \cdot 100$$

STEP 6. Write the whole number 100 in fraction form.

$$\frac{5}{2}x = \frac{4}{25} \cdot \frac{100}{1}$$

STEP 7. To obtain 1x, multiply both sides by $\frac{2}{5}$, the reciprocal of $\frac{5}{2}$.

$$\frac{2}{5} \cdot \frac{5}{2}x = \frac{4}{25} \cdot \frac{100}{1} \cdot \frac{2}{5}$$

STEP 8. Cross cancel.

$$\frac{\overset{1}{\cancel{2}}}{\underset{1}{\cancel{5}}} \cdot \frac{\overset{1}{\cancel{5}}}{\underset{1}{\cancel{2}}}x = \frac{4}{\underset{1}{25}} \cdot \frac{\overset{4}{\cancel{100}}}{1} \cdot \frac{2}{5}$$

STEP 9. Multiply.

$$x = \frac{32}{5}$$

STEP 10. Change the improper fraction to a mixed number.

$$x = 6\frac{2}{5}$$

The answer is $6\frac{2}{5}$.

Or you can solve the problem this way:

Example 6: $2\frac{1}{2}\%$ of what is 0.16?

STEP 1. Write $2\frac{1}{2}$ as a decimal number.

$$2\frac{1}{2} = 2\frac{5}{10} = 2.5$$

STEP 2. Rewrite the problem.

2.5% of what is 0.16?

STEP 3. Substitute the given information into the percent proportion.

$$\frac{0.16}{x} \times \frac{2.5}{100}$$

STEP 4. Cross multiply and place the variable on the left side of the equation.

$$2.5x = 0.16 \cdot 100$$

STEP 5. Divide both sides by the number to the left of the x.

$$\frac{^1\cancel{2.5}x}{_1\cancel{2.5}} = \frac{16}{2.5}$$

$$x = 6.4$$

$$2.5\overline{)16.0.0}^{\;6.4}$$

The answer is 6.4.

Tip: Examples 5 and 6 illustrate two different ways to solve a percent proportion problem that contains both a fraction and a decimal number. Notice that you need fewer steps when using two decimal numbers than when using two fractions. However, long division with decimal numbers can be very tedious. If you know the fraction rules, the fraction method is actually faster. You need to decide which method works best for you.

4.2 Practice the Percent Proportion

Solve the following problems. For the answers, see "Step-by-Step Solutions" (pages 259 to 262). Use the percent proportion to solve each problem.

1. 30% of 60 is what?

2. 7 = what % of 35?

3. 70 is 20% of what?

4. 3.2% of 47 is what?

5. What is 150% of 52?

6. 0.4% of 80 is what?

7. $\frac{3}{5}$ is what % of 2?

8. 7 is 35% of what number?

9. What percent of 614 is 135.08?

10. 979.2 is 54.4% of what number?

11. $37\frac{1}{2}$% of what is 61.2?

12. 16.2 is what percent of 45?

13. 35% of 22.4 is what?

14. What percent of 49 is 34.3?

15. 119.6 is 23% of what number?

16. What number is 12% of 700?

17. 9.5 is 25% of what?

18. 3 is $\frac{5}{9}$ % of what?

19. 33 is 16.5% of what?

20. $66\frac{3}{5}$ is what percent of 360?

In this section, we will review:
- changing a percent to a fraction
- changing a fraction to a percent
- changing a ratio to a percent

Changing a Percent to a Fraction

These are the steps for changing a percent to a fraction:

1. Remove the percent sign.
2. Write the number over 100. Now you have the fraction form.
3. Write the fraction in reduced form. (See Section 2.1, Lowest Terms and Reduced Form, page 20.)

Example 1:   Write 25% as a fraction.

STEP 1. Remove the percent sign.   **25**

STEP 2. Write the number over 100. $\dfrac{25}{100}$

STEP 3. Write the fraction in reduced form. $\dfrac{\cancel{25}^{1}}{\cancel{100}_{4}} = \dfrac{1}{4}$

The answer is $\dfrac{1}{4}$.

Example 2:   Change 12% to a reduced fraction.

STEP 1. Remove the percent sign.   **12**

STEP 2. Write the number over 100. $\dfrac{12}{100}$

STEP 3. Write the fraction in reduced form. $\dfrac{\cancel{12}^{3}}{\cancel{100}_{25}} = \dfrac{3}{25}$

The answer is $\dfrac{3}{25}$.

Example 3: Write 37.5% as a fraction.

STEP 1. First remove the percent sign.

$$37.5$$

STEP 2. Write the number over 100.

$$\frac{37.5}{100}$$

STEP 3. Multiply the decimal number in the numerator by a power of 10 to make it a whole number. Multiply the denominator by the same power of 10 to form equivalent fractions.

$$\frac{37.5}{100} \cdot \frac{10}{10} = \frac{375}{1,000}$$

STEP 4. Write the fraction in reduced form.

$$\frac{\overset{3}{\cancel{\overset{75}{\cancel{375}}}}}{\underset{\underset{8}{\cancel{200}}}{\cancel{1,000}}} = \frac{3}{8}$$

The answer is $\frac{3}{8}$.

Your work should look like this on paper.

$$37.5\% = \frac{37.5}{100} \cdot \frac{10}{10} = \frac{\overset{3}{\cancel{\overset{75}{\cancel{375}}}}}{\underset{\underset{8}{\cancel{200}}}{\cancel{1,000}}} = \frac{3}{8}$$

Changing a Fraction to a Percent

Remember that percent can be shown as $\frac{x}{100}$.

These are the steps for changing a fraction to a percent:

1. Set the fraction equal to $\frac{x}{100}$
2. Solve the proportion.
3. Write the answer as a percent.

Example 4: Write $\frac{1}{5}$ as a percent.

STEP 1. Set the fraction equal to $\frac{x}{100}$.

$$\frac{1}{5} = \frac{x}{100}$$

STEP 2. Solve the proportion.

$$5x = 100$$

$$\frac{\cancel{5}x}{\cancel{5}} = \frac{100}{5}$$

$$5)\overline{100} \quad \frac{20}{}$$

$$x = 20$$

STEP 3. Write the answer as a percent.

$$x = 20\%$$

The answer is 20%.

Example 5: Write $\frac{32}{25}$ as a percent.

STEP 1. Set the fraction equal to $\frac{x}{100}$.

$$\frac{32}{25} = \frac{x}{100}$$

STEP 2. Solve the proportion.

$$25x = 3,200$$

$$\frac{\cancel{25}x}{\cancel{25}} = \frac{3,200}{25}$$

$$25)\overline{3,200} \quad \frac{128}{}$$

$$x = 128$$

STEP 3. Write the answer as a percent.

$$x = 128\%$$

The answer is 128%.

Changing a Ratio to a Percent

Changing a ratio to a percent is very similar to changing a fraction to a percent. It requires one additional step. These are the steps for changing a ratio to a percent:

1. Write the ratio in fraction form.
2. Set the fraction equal to $\frac{x}{100}$.
3. Solve the proportion.
4. Write the answer as a percent.

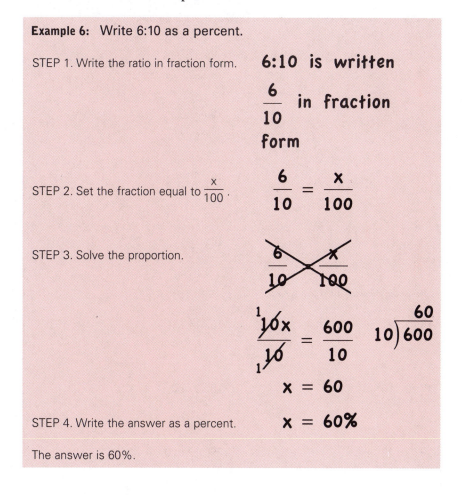

Example 6: Write 6:10 as a percent.

STEP 1. Write the ratio in fraction form.

6:10 is written $\frac{6}{10}$ in fraction form

STEP 2. Set the fraction equal to $\frac{x}{100}$.

$$\frac{6}{10} = \frac{x}{100}$$

STEP 3. Solve the proportion.

$$\frac{\cancel{6}}{\cancel{10}} \diagdown \frac{\cancel{x}}{\cancel{100}}$$

$$\frac{\cancel{10}^1 x}{\cancel{10}_1} = \frac{600}{10} \qquad 10\overline{)600}^{\;60}$$

$$x = 60$$

STEP 4. Write the answer as a percent.

$$x = 60\%$$

The answer is 60%.

4.3 Practice Fractions, Ratios, and Percents

Solve the following problems. For the answers, see "Step-by-Step Solutions" (pages 262 to 264). Change the following percents to a reduced fraction.

1. Write 50% as a fraction.

2. Write 74.25% as a fraction.

3. Write 12.5% as a fraction.

4. Write 60% as a fraction.

5. Write 165% as a mixed number.

6. Write 45.375% as a fraction.

Change the following fractions to a percent. Use the percent proportion.

7. $\dfrac{1}{2}$

8. $\dfrac{19}{10}$

9. $\dfrac{2}{3}$

10. $\dfrac{1}{6}$

11. $\dfrac{11}{8}$

12. $\dfrac{3}{5}$

13. $\dfrac{7}{25}$

14. $\dfrac{7}{4}$

Change the following ratios to a percent.

15. 3 : 8

16. 14 : 30

17. 9 : 10

18. 2 : 50

19. 3 : 25

20. 12 : 20

Working with Percents and Decimal Numbers

In this section, we will review:
- changing a decimal number to a percent
- changing a percent to a decimal number
- performing computations with a % sign

Changing a Decimal Number to a Percent

These are the steps for changing a decimal to a percent:

1. Move the decimal point two places to the right. This is the same as multiplying by 100.
2. Write the resulting number.
3. Place a percent (%) sign after the number.

Example 1: Change 0.05 to a percent.

STEP 1. Move the decimal point two places to the right. **0.05.**

STEP 2. Write the resulting number. **5**

STEP 3. Write a percent sign after the number. **5%**

The answer is 5%.

Your work should look like this on paper.

0.05 = 0.05. = 5%

Example 2: Change 3.49 to a percent.

STEP 1. Move the decimal point two places to the right. **3.49.**

STEP 2. Write the resulting number. **349**

STEP 3. Write a percent sign after the number. **349%**

The answer is 349%.

Your work should look like this on paper.

3.49 = 3.49. = 349%

Example 3: Change 7 to a percent.

STEP 1. Move the decimal point two places to the right.   **7.00.**

STEP 2. Write the resulting number.   **700**

STEP 3. Write a percent sign after the number.   **700%**

The answer is 700%.

Your work should look like this on paper.

$$7 = 7.00. = 700\%$$

Changing a Percent to a Decimal

To change a percent to a decimal follow these steps.

1. Remove the percent sign.
2. Move the decimal point two places to the left. This is same as dividing by 100.
3. Place a zero to the left of the decimal point, if needed.
4. Remove any trailing zeros, if needed.

Example 4: Change 25% to a decimal number.

STEP 1. Remove the percent sign.   **25**

STEP 2. Move the decimal point 2 places to the left.   **.25.**

STEP 3. Place a zero to the left of the decimal point.   **0.25**

The answer is 0.25.

Your work should look like this on paper.

$$25\% = .25. = 0.25$$

Example 5: Change 2% to a decimal number.

STEP 1. Remove the percent sign.   **2**

STEP 2. Move the decimal point 2 places to the left.   **.02.**

STEP 3. Place a zero to the left of the decimal point.   **0.02**

The answer is 0.02.

Your work should look like this on paper.

$$2\% \ = \ .02. \ = \ 0.02$$

Example 6: Change 100% to a decimal number.

STEP 1. Remove the percent sign.   **100**

STEP 2. Move the decimal point 2 places to the left.   **1.00.**

STEP 3. Remove the trailing zeros.   **1.00**

The answer is 1.   **1**

Your work should look like this on paper.

$$100\% \ = \ 1.00. \ = \ 1$$

Example 7: Change 230% to a decimal number.

STEP 1. Remove the percent sign.   **230**

STEP 2. Move the decimal point 2 places to the left.   **2.30.**
This is the same as dividing by 100.

STEP 3. Remove the trailing zero.   **2.30**

The answer is 2.3.   **2.3**

Your work should look like this on paper.

$$230\% \ = \ 2.30. \ = \ 2.30 \ = \ 2.3$$

Tip: Here is an easy way to remember which direction to move the decimal point when changing a decimal number to a percent or changing a percent to a decimal number. Think of the alphabet:

ABCDEFGHIJKLMNOPQRSTUVWXYZ

Write the letters D and P.

D stands for decimal number.

P stands for percent.

1. To get from *D* to *P* in the alphabet, move right: D⇨P.
   So, to change a Decimal number to a Percent, move the decimal point to the right: Decimal⇨Percent.

2. To get from *P* to *D* in the alphabet, move left: D⇦P.
   So, to change a Percent to a Decimal number, move the decimal point to the left: Decimal⇦Percent.

Performing Computations with a % Sign

Percents can be added or subtracted. For example, 65% + 20% = 85% and 50% - 10% = 40%. However, the percent form of a number, such as 75%, must be written as a decimal number, 0.75, before performing multiplication or division.

These are the steps for solving a multiplication or division problem containing a % sign:

1. Change the term containing the % sign to a decimal number.
2. Rewrite the problem with the decimal number.
3. Multiply or divide to solve the problem.

Example 8: $\dfrac{130}{40\%}$

STEP 1. Change the percent to a decimal number. Remove any trailing zeros.

$$40\% = .40. = 0.40 = 0.4$$

STEP 2. Rewrite the problem with the decimal number.

$$\frac{130}{0.4}$$

STEP 3. Divide to solve the problem. (See Section 3.5, Dividing Decimal Numbers, page 75.)

$$0.4.\overline{)130.0.} \quad \begin{array}{r} 32\ 5. \\ \end{array} = 325$$

The answer is 325.

Your work should look like this on paper.

$$\frac{130}{40\%} = \frac{130}{.40.} = \frac{130}{0.40} = \frac{130}{0.4} = 325$$

4.4 Practice Percents and Decimal Numbers

Solve the following problems. For the answers, see "Step-by-Step Solutions" (pages 264 to 265).
Change each decimal number to a percent.

1. 0.02   **2.** 0.7

3. 2.575   **4.** 3

5. 1.43   **6.** 0.185

7. 0.308

Change each percent to a decimal number.

8. 25%   **9.** 1%

10. 130%   **11.** 52.5%

12. 88%   **13.** 425%

14. 75.25%

Solve the following division problems.

15. $\dfrac{153}{45\%}$

16. $\dfrac{4.4}{20\%}$

17. $\dfrac{150}{40\%}$

18. $\dfrac{2.7}{45\%}$

19. $\dfrac{6.48}{36\%}$

20. $\dfrac{20}{100\%}$

4.5

Fraction, Decimal, and Percent Table
In this section, we will review:
- common fractions written as decimal numbers and percents
- fractions that require speedy recall

Common Equivalents

Fractions, decimals, and percents are all used in the nursing profession. For speedy recall, memorize the commonly used fractions, decimals, and percents shown in Table 4.1: Commonly Used Equivalents for Fractions, Decimals, and Percents.

Table 4.1	Commonly Used Equivalents for Fractions, Decimals, and Percents		
	Fraction	Decimal	Percent
ONE-HALF	$\dfrac{1}{2}$	0.5	50%
THIRDS	$\dfrac{1}{3}$	0.33... or $0.\overline{3}$	$33\dfrac{1}{3}\%$
	$\dfrac{2}{3}$	0.66... or $0.\overline{6}$	$66\dfrac{2}{3}\%$

Table 4.1	Commonly Used Equivalents for Fractions, Decimals, and Percents—cont'd		
	Fraction	Decimal	Percent
FOURTHS or QUARTERS	$\frac{1}{4}$	0.25	25%
	$\frac{3}{4}$	0.75	75%
FIFTHS	$\frac{1}{5}$	0.2	20%
	$\frac{2}{5}$	0.4	40%
	$\frac{3}{5}$	0.6	60%
	$\frac{4}{5}$	0.8	80%
EIGHTHS	$\frac{1}{8}$	0.125	12.5%
	$\frac{3}{8}$	0.375	37.5%
	$\frac{5}{8}$	0.625	62.5%
	$\frac{7}{8}$	0.875	87.5%
TENTHS	$\frac{1}{10}$	0.1	10%
	$\frac{3}{10}$	0.3	30%
	$\frac{7}{10}$	0.7	70%
	$\frac{9}{10}$	0.9	90%

Chapter Test for Percents, Ratios, and Proportions

Solve the following problems. After taking the test, see "Step-by-Step Solutions" for the answers (pages 265 to 268). And see "4.1 Ratios and Proportions," " 4.2 The Percent Proportion," "4.3 Fractions, Ratios, and Percents," and "4.4 Working with Percents and Decimal Numbers," if the chapter test indicates you need additional practice.

Section 4.1

Solve each proportion for x.

1. $\dfrac{2}{5} = \dfrac{x}{45}$

2. $\dfrac{x}{4} = \dfrac{36}{23}$

Section 4.2

Write the percent proportion to solve for x.

3. x is 25% of 24.

4. 125 is what percent of 37.5?

5. 139.6 is 20% of x.

6. $\dfrac{4}{5}$ % of x is 5.

7. $\dfrac{1}{2}$ is what percent of $\dfrac{5}{4}$?

8. 12.5% of 600 is what number?

Section 4.3

Change each % to a fraction in reduced form.

9. 15%

10. 62.5%

Write each fraction as a percent.

11. Write $\dfrac{9}{5}$ as a percent.

12. Write $\dfrac{1}{3}$ as a percent.

Write the ratio as a percent.

13. 7:20

Section 4.4

Change each percent to a decimal number.

14. 100%   **15.** 37.5%

Change each decimal number to a percent.

16. 3.49   **17.** 7

Solve.

18. $\dfrac{32}{20\%}$ **19.** $\dfrac{150}{10\%}$ **20.** $\dfrac{50}{100\%}$

Positive and Negative Numbers

chapter 5

5.0 Pretest for Positive and Negative Numbers

Solve the following problems. After taking the test, see "Step-by-Step Solutions" for the answers (page 269). Then, see "5.1 Adding Positive and Negative Numbers," "5.2 Subtracting Positive and Negative Numbers," "5.3 Multiplying and Dividing Positive and Negative Numbers," "5.4 Collecting Like Terms," and "5.5 The Distributive Property" for skill explanations.

Section 5.1

1. $(-14) + (-9)$

2. $28 + (-13)$

Section 5.2

3. $17 - (-8)$

4. $3 - 27$

Section 5.3

5. $3(-8)$

6. $\dfrac{-56}{-8}$

Section 5.4

7. $x^2 + 3x - 1 - 3x^2 + 4$

8. $3x^4 + 2x^4 - 7 - 25$

Section 5.5

9. $3(-2y - 7)$

10. $-(-x^2 + 5x - 9)$

Adding Positive and Negative Numbers
In this section, we will review:
- the number line
- positive and negative numbers
- rules for adding positive and negative numbers

The Number Line

Positive and negative numbers as well as the addition of positive and negative numbers are easily illustrated on a **number line**. (See Fig. 5.1.)

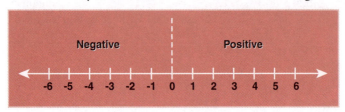

Figure 5.1: Visualizing negative and positive numbers.

Positive and Negative Numbers

Positive numbers are greater than zero and are located to the right of zero on a number line. Positive numbers get larger as you move to the right on a number line. They can be written with or without a positive sign (+). In **best mathematical form**, positive numbers do not have the + sign in front of them. All of these numbers indicate positive numbers: 1, +1; 2, +2; and 3, +3.

Negative numbers are less than zero and are located to the left of zero on a number line. Negative numbers get smaller as you move to the left on the number line. They are written with a negative sign (−). If a negative number is part of a problem, keep the entire number in a parenthesis. The number should look like this: (−2) + (−7). For an answer, a negative number is not written in parenthesis. These numbers indicate negative answers: −1, −2, and −3.

Rules for Adding Positive and Negative Numbers

There are three rules for adding positive and negative numbers. Memorize the rules.

Rule 1: The sum of two positive numbers is a positive number. For example, $1 + 1 = 2$. (See Fig. 5.2.)

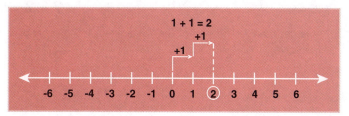

Figure 5.2: The sum of two positive numbers.

Rule 2: The sum of two negative numbers is a negative number. For example, $(-1) + (-1) = -2$. When you add two negatives, note that the answer is on the negative side of the number line. (See Fig. 5.3.)

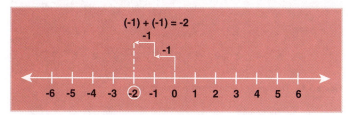

Figure 5.3: The sum of two negative numbers.

Rule 3: The sum of a positive number plus a negative number can be either positive or negative. The answer depends on the sign of the larger number. Therefore, to find the sum of a **positive number** and a **negative number** follow these steps:

1. Look only at the numbers, not their signs. **Subtract the two numbers**. Do not worry about whether they are positive or negative numbers.
2. **Use the sign of the larger number** for your answer.

Example 1: 2 + (–7)

STEP 1. Look at only the numbers, not their signs.

STEP 2. Subtract.

STEP 3. 7 is larger than 2. The sign of the 7 is a – (negative).

The answer is –5.

Your work should look like this on paper.

$$2 + (-7)$$
$$7 - 2 = 5$$
$$-5$$

$$2 + (-7) = -5$$

If you use a number line to solve this problem, you will get the same answer. (See Fig. 5.4.)

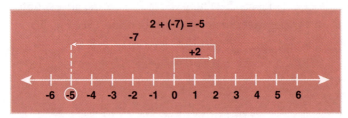

Figure 5.4: The sum of a positive and a negative number.

Example 2: (–6) + 8

STEP 1. Look only at the numbers, not their signs.

STEP 2. Subtract.

STEP 3. Notice that 8 is larger than 6. The sign of the 8 is positive.

The answer is +2, written 2.

Your work should look like this on paper.

$$(-6) + 8$$
$$8 - 6 = 2$$
$$2$$

$$(-6) + 8 = 2$$

Rule 4: Any positive number added to its opposite (the negative) is 0: $5 + (-5) = 0$. This is the way a problem looks on a number line. (See Fig. 5.5.)

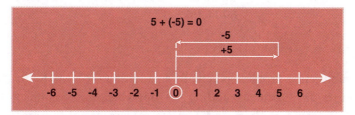

Figure 5.5: A positive number added to its negative number.

5.1 Practice Adding Positive and Negative Numbers

Solve the following problems. For the answers, see "Step-by-Step Solutions" (pages 270 to 271).

1. $(-5) + 30$ 2. $(-8) + 6$ 3. $(-9) + (-15)$

4. $30 + 5$ 5. $(-8) + (-8)$ 6. $40 + (-20)$

7. $(-9) + 5$ 8. $7 + (-10)$ 9. $25 + 15$

10. $8 + (-9)$ 11. $(-42) + (-36)$ 12. $15 + 30$

13. $4 + (-4)$ 14. $10 + (-20)$ 15. $4 + (-2)$

16. $6 + (-7)$ 17. $(-5) + 9$ 18. $(-1) + (-1)$

19. $(-14) + (-7)$ 20. $(-1,234) + 1,234$

Subtracting Positive and Negative Numbers
In this section, we will review:
- rewriting subtraction as addition
- the rules for adding positive and negative numbers

Rewriting Subtraction as Addition

Every subtraction problem is actually an addition problem. **Subtracting a number is the same as adding its opposite.** For example, **5 – 4** means the same as **5 + (–4)**. The answers are the same whether you write the problem as subtraction or addition: **5 – 4 = 1** and **5 + (–4) = 1**.

These are the three steps for changing a subtraction problem to an addition problem:

1. Change the subtraction sign to addition.
2. Write the opposite of the number that follows the subtraction sign.
3. After rewriting subtraction as addition, apply the rules for adding positive and negative numbers.

Example 1:   10 – 7

STEP 1. Change the subtraction sign to addition.

10 +

STEP 2. Write the opposite of the number that follows the subtraction sign.

10 + (–7)

STEP 3. Apply the rules for adding a positive and negative number. Look only at the numbers, not their signs. Subtract: 10 – 7 = 3. Since 10 is larger than 7, the sign of the 3 is positive.

3

The answer is +3, written 3.

Your work should look like this on paper. **10 – 7**
10 + (–7)
3

Example 2: $7 - 9$

STEP 1. Change the subtraction sign to addition. $7 +$

STEP 2. Write the opposite of the number that follows the subtraction sign. $7 + (-9)$

STEP 3. Apply the rules for adding a positive and negative number. Look only at the numbers, not their signs. Subtract: $9 - 7 = 2$. Since 9 is larger than 7, the sign of the 2 is negative. -2

The answer is -2.

Your work should look like this on paper. $7 - 9$
$$7 + (-9)$$
$$-2$$

Example 3: $(-7) - 14$

STEP 1. Change the subtraction sign to addition. $(-7) +$

STEP 2. Write the opposite of the number that follows the subtraction sign. $(-7) + (-14)$

STEP 3. Apply the rule for adding two negative numbers. The sum of two negative numbers is a negative number. -21

The answer is -21.

Your work should look like this on paper. $(-7) - 14$
$$(-7) + (-14)$$
$$-21$$

Example 4: $(-4) - (-21)$

STEP 1. Change the subtraction sign to addition.

$$(-4) +$$

STEP 2. Write the opposite of the number that follows the subtraction sign.

$$(-4) + 21$$

STEP 3. Apply the rules for adding a positive and negative number. Look only at the numbers, not their signs. Subtract: $21 - 4 = 17$. Since 21 is larger than 4, the sign of the 17 is positive.

$$17$$

The answer is 17.

Your work should look like this on paper.

$$(-4) - (-21)$$
$$(-4) + 21$$
$$17$$

Example 5: $8 - (-3)$

STEP 1. Change the subtraction sign to addition.

$$8 +$$

STEP 2. Write the opposite of the number that follows the subtraction sign.

$$8 + 3$$

STEP 3. Apply the rule for adding two positive numbers. The sum of two positive numbers is a positive number. $8 + 3 = 11$.

$$11$$

The answer is 11.

Your work should look like this on paper.

$$8 - (-3)$$
$$8 + 3$$
$$11$$

5.2 Practice Subtracting Positive and Negative Numbers

Solve the following problems. For the answers, see "Step-by-Step Solutions" (pages 271 to 272).

Rewrite subtraction problems as addition problems. Use the rules for adding positive and negative integers. Then solve.

1. 31 – 12

2. 8 – 79

3. 11 – 46

4. (–15) – 65

5. 14 – (–8)

6. (–19) – 17

7. (–7) – (–31)

8. 12 – (–63)

9. (–61) – (–5)

10. 69 – 18

11. (–9) – 7

12. (–47) – (–28)

13. 47 – 58

14. (–9) – (–10)

15. (–19) – 5

16. (–16) – (–18)

17. 31 – 17

18. (–11) – 6

19. 99 – (–1)

20. (–8) – (–12)

**Multiplying and Dividing Positive
and Negative Numbers**
In this section, we will review:
- a new way to indicate multiplication
- rules for multiplying positive and negative
  numbers
- rules for dividing positive and negative
  numbers

A New Way to Indicate Multiplication

Parentheses indicate multiplication. For example,

$$3(9) = 27 \qquad (4)(5) = 20$$

Rules for Multiplying Positive and Negative Numbers

There are three rules for multiplying positive and negative numbers. Memorize the rules.

Rule 1: The product of two positive numbers is a positive number. For example:

**positive • positive = positive
7 • 8 = 56**

Rule 2: The product of two negative numbers is a positive number. For example:

**negative • negative = positive
(-9)(-6) = 54**

Rule 3: The product of a positive number and a negative number is negative. For example:

**positive • negative = negative
6(-3) = -18**

**negative • positive = negative
-3(4) = -12**

Rules for Dividing Positive and Negative Numbers

The rules for dividing positive and negative numbers are the same as the rules for multiplying except that you divide rather than multiply. For example,

Rule 1:

$$\frac{\text{positive (+)}}{\text{positive (+)}} = \text{positive (+)}$$

$$\frac{6}{3} = 2$$

Rule 2:

$$\frac{\text{negative (-)}}{\text{negative (-)}} = \text{positive (+)}$$

$$\frac{-8}{-2} = 4$$

Rule 3:

$$\frac{\text{positive (+)}}{\text{negative (-)}} = \text{negative (-)}$$

$$\frac{12}{-36} = -\frac{1}{3}$$

$$\frac{\text{negative (-)}}{\text{positive (+)}} = \text{negative (-)}$$

$$\frac{-27}{6} = -\frac{9}{2}$$

If the final answer is an improper fraction, reduce it. Then write the answer as an improper fraction (not a mixed number).

5.3 Practice Multiplying and Dividing Positive and Negative Numbers

Solve the following problems. For the answers, see "Step-by-Step Solutions" (page 272).

1. $(-9)(1)$

2. $5(-1)$

3. $(-10)(-4)$

4. $(-7)(-4)$

5. $(-5)(-2)$

6. $(-2)(-4)$

7. $6(-8)$

8. $5(-4)$

9. $(-14)(0)$

10. $8(4)$

11. $\dfrac{-77}{7}$

12. $\dfrac{81}{9}$

13. $\dfrac{-24}{-2}$

14. $\dfrac{48}{-6}$

15. $\dfrac{72}{-8}$

16. $\dfrac{-14}{-2}$

17. $\dfrac{-36}{6}$

18. $\dfrac{45}{-9}$

19. $\dfrac{35}{-5}$

20. $\dfrac{56}{8}$

Collecting Like Terms

In this section, we will review:
- terminology for algebra
- collecting like terms

Terminology for Algebra

In algebra, we often use letters as **variables** to take the place of numbers. For example, in—

5x, x is the variable.

-4y, y is the variable.

A **coefficient** is the number that you see to the left of a variable (letter). For example, in—

4xy, 4 is the coefficient.

-5y, -5 is the coefficient.

z, 1 is the coefficient.

The coefficient is always understood to be 1 when a number does not appear to the left of the variable (letter).

An **expression** is a mathematical statement that may contain numbers, variables, or both. For example,

-9y and **8x + 7** are expressions.

Exponents, also known as **powers,** indicate how many times a variable (letter) or number is multiplied by itself. For example,

5^2 means **5 • 5**. The small ^{2} is the exponent. And 5^2 is read either 5 raised to the second power or 5 squared.

Collecting Like Terms

Term in math means one part of an algebraic expression. A term may be a number, a variable, or a product of both. For example, the expression **$7x^2 + 4x - 9$** has three terms. They are **$7x^2$**, **+4x**, and **-9**.

Like terms contain the same variable raised to the same power. The coefficients of like terms are different.

In these groups of numbers,

5x and **-4x** are like terms.

$3xy^2$ and **$15xy^2$** are like terms.

4 and **-9** are like terms because they are numbers (**constants**).

In these expressions, the like terms appear as **underlined, boxed, or circled.**

$$\underline{4x}\ \boxed{-\,3y^2}\ \textcircled{$+7$}\ \underline{-\,2x}\ \boxed{-\,5y^2}\ \textcircled{$+\,4$}$$

$$\underline{3x^2y} - \underline{7x^2y} + 10xy^2\ \boxed{+\,15}\ \boxed{-\,9}$$

To **collect like terms**, identify the terms that have the same variable raised to the same power. Then add or subtract the like terms using the rules for adding and subtracting positive and negative numbers.

When you add or subtract like terms, change only the coefficient (the number in front of the variable). The variable remains the same. For example,

$$8x - 6x = 2x$$

$$-9y^2 + 2y^2 = -7y^2$$

$$5xy^2 - xy^2 = 4xy^2$$

In algebra, the **order of operations** is specific. The rule for addition and subtraction is to work from left to right, adding and subtracting terms as you come to them.

Tip: When collecting like terms, keep in mind that subtracting a number is the same as adding its opposite. Then apply the rules for adding positive and negative numbers as you collect the like terms.

To solve an algebraic expression follow these steps.

1. Identify and mark like terms by underlining, circling, or drawing boxes around them.
2. Starting with the first term in the expression, add all like terms to the right in the order in which they appear. Remember to use the rules for adding positive and negative numbers. Write that sum as the first term in the answer. Cross out terms after adding them.
3. If there are no like terms, write the term in the answer, cross out the term, and move to the next term.
4. Repeat this process, always beginning with the first remaining term on the left side of the expression. Continue until all terms have been marked out.

Example 1: $6x^2 + 8 - 9x^2 + 2$

STEP 1. Identify and mark like terms by underlining, circling, or drawing boxes around them.

$$\underline{6x^2}\ \boxed{+8}\ -\underline{9x^2}\ \boxed{+2}$$

STEP 2. Starting with the first term in the expression, add the like terms.

$$6x^2 + (-9x^2) = -3x^2$$

STEP 3. Write $-3x^2$ as the first term in the answer.

STEP 4. Cross out $6x^2$ and $-9x^2$.

$$\cancel{6x^2} + 8\ \cancel{-9x^2} + 2$$

STEP 5. Go back to the left side of the expression, and add the next like terms.

$$8 + 2 = 10$$

STEP 6. Write 10 as the second term in the answer.

STEP 7. Cross out $+8$ and $+2$.

$$\cancel{6x^2} + \cancel{8}\ \cancel{-9x^2} + \cancel{2}$$

The answer is $-3x^2 + 10$.

$$-3x^2 + 10$$

Your work should look like this on paper.

$$\cancel{\underline{6x^2}}\ \boxed{+8}\ \cancel{-\underline{9x^2}}\ \boxed{+2} = -3x^2 + 10$$

Example 2: $4x - 3y^2 + 9xy + 7 - 2x - 5y^2 + 4$

STEP 1. Identify the like terms. Mark them by underlining, circling, or drawing boxes.

$$\underline{4x}\ \boxed{-3y^2} + 9xy\ \boxed{+7}\ \underline{-2x}\ \boxed{-5y^2}\ \boxed{+4}$$

STEP 2. Starting with the first term in the expression, add the like terms.

$$4x + (-2x) = 2x$$

STEP 3. Write $2x$ as the first term in your answer.

STEP 4. Cross out $4x$ and $-2x$.

$$\cancel{4x} - 3y^2 + 9xy + 7\ \cancel{-2x} - 5y^2 + 4$$

STEP 5. Go back to the left side of the expression, and add the next like terms.

$$-3y^2 + (-5y^2) = -8y^2$$

STEP 6. Write $-8y^2$ as the second term in your answer.

STEP 7. Cross out $-3y^2$ and $-5y^2$.

$$4x\ \cancel{-3y^2} + 9xy + 7\ -2x\ \cancel{-5y^2} + 4$$

STEP 8. Go back to the left side of the expression. Look at the next term, $+9xy$. There is no like term for $+9xy$. Cross out $+9xy$. Write it as the third term in your answer and move to the next term.

$$\cancel{4x}\ \cancel{-3y^2}\ \cancel{+9xy} + 7\ \cancel{-2x}\ \cancel{-5y^2} + 4$$

STEP 9. Look at the term to the right of $9xy$. It is $+7$. So, add $+7$ and $+4$.

$$7 + 4 = 11$$

STEP 10. Write 11 as the fourth term in the answer.

STEP 11. Cross out $+7$ and $+4$.

$$\cancel{4x}\ \cancel{-3y^2}\ \cancel{+9xy}\ \cancel{+7}\ \cancel{-2x}\ \cancel{-5y^2}\ \cancel{+4}$$

The answer is $2x - 8y^2 + 9xy + 11$.

$$2x - 8y^2 + 9xy + 11$$

Your work should look like this on paper.

$$\cancel{4x}\ \boxed{-3y^2}\ \cancel{+9xy}\ \boxed{+7}\ \cancel{-2x}\ \boxed{-5y^2}\ \boxed{+4} = 2x - 8y^2 + 9xy + 11$$

Tip: Sometimes, the order of the terms in your answer may not match a choice on a test. To find the correct choice, look at each term in your answer. Choose the answer that has the same terms including any positive or negative signs.

For example, these answers all have the same meaning:

$$2x - 8y^2 + 9xy + 11$$
$$-8y^2 + 2x + 9xy + 11$$
$$2x - 8y^2 + 11 + 9xy$$

5.4 Practice Collecting Like Terms

Solve the following problems. For the answers, see "Step-by-Step Solutions" (pages 272 to 273).
Collect like terms. Use the rules for adding and subtracting positive and negative numbers..

1. $4y - 8y$

2. $(-9x) - 4x$

3. $-5b + 4b$

4. $5bx^2 - 2bx^2$

5. $x - 8x$

6. $(-6x) + 6x$

7. $5a + 2a^2 + 6a$

8. $4y + 3y - 2xy$

9. $3a^2 + 4a^2 + 5$

10. $-45a + 44a$

11. $2x - 3 + 3x - 2$

12. $6a^2 + 7a^2 + 8$

13. $3a - 1 + a + 3b$

14. $-a + 2 + 8a^2 - 7$

15. $-4x^2 + 8 - 5xy + 2x^2 - 10$

16. $-9x - x^2 + x - 2x^2 + 4$

17. $-18a^2 + 17a^2$

18. $(-5x) + 6 - 3x$

19. $7a^3 + 3 - 7a^3 - 3$

20. $-6x^2 - 1 - x - 10$

The Distributive Property

In this section, we will review:
- another use of parentheses in multiplication
- the distributive property

Another Use of Parentheses in Multiplication

Parentheses can mean to multiply numbers, for example 4(5), as well as to multiply expressions containing numbers and variables, for example 4(5x). However, an expression such as $4(x + y)$ indicates two operations are needed: multiplication and addition. To simplify $4(x + y)$, you need to use the distributive property.

The Distributive Property

The distributive property states that $a(b + c) = ab + ac$ or $a(b − c) = ab − ac$.

In other words, each term within the parentheses is multiplied by the value to the left of the parentheses. **When you apply the distributive property, the rules for multiplying positive and negative numbers are in force.**

Let's look at $4(x + y)$. You cannot add x and y because you do not know the value of x or y. However, you can use the distributive property to multiply 4 times x and to multiply 4 times y. Then, you can show the two products, 4x and 4y, as the sum $4x + 4y$.

$$4(x + y) = 4x + 4y$$

Tip: Think of the distributive property process as being similar to dealing cards. You take the number on the outside of the parentheses, and deal it to each term inside the parentheses.

You can use the distributive property to multiply any number of terms in parentheses. The resulting answer will have the same number of terms as are in the parentheses. For example,

$$5(r + 2) = 5r + 10$$
$$-4(5a + 6) = -20a - 24$$

$$\overset{\frown}{3(2x} \overset{\frown}{- 9)} = 6x - 27$$

$$\overset{\frown}{-2(x^{2}} \overset{\frown}{+ 3x} \overset{\frown}{- 4)} = -2x^{2} - 6x + 8$$

If a negative sign is to the left of the parentheses, like $-(a + 4)$, then it is understood that -1 is in front of the parenthesis. Distribute -1 to both terms, then simplify. For example,

$$\overset{\frown}{-1(a} \overset{\frown}{+ 4)}$$
$$-1(a) + (-1)(4)$$
$$-a + (-4)$$
$$-a - 4$$

5.5 Practice The Distributive Property

Solve the following problems using the distributive property. For the answers, see "Step-by-Step Solutions" (pages 273 to 274).

1. $5(2x + 1)$
2. $2(-4x - 3)$
3. $-7(-3y + 2)$

4. $-3(5x^2 + 4x - 7)$
5. $-3(2x^2 + x - 4)$
6. $-4(-3x + 2)$

7. $-(a + 1)$
8. $-8(2a + 3)$
9. $-4(-x - 5)$

10. $-7(4x^2 - 5x - 2)$
11. $-9(2 - y)$
12. $-(2x + 5)$

13. $2(-x^3 + x^2 - 1)$
14. $-3(x - 2)$
15. $-(y - 2)$

16. $-(-y + 5)$
17. $3(x + y + 5)$
18. $-4(5y + 6x - 2)$

19. $-2(x^2 + 3x - 4)$
20. $-(3x + 7y + 9)$

Solve the following problems. After taking the test, see "Step-by-Step Solutions" for the answers (pages 274 to 275). And see "5.1 Adding Positive and Negative Numbers," "5.2 Subtracting Positive and Negative Numbers," "5.3 Multiplying and Dividing Positive and Negative Numbers," "5.4 Collecting Like Terms," and "5.5 The Distributive Property" if the chapter test indicates you need additional practice.

Section 5.1

1. $-6 + 12$

2. $-18 + 18$

3. $6 + (-4)$

4. $-5 + (-29)$

Section 5.2

5. $32 - 13$

6. $(-8) - (-6)$

7. $9 - 81$

8. $(-14) - 67$

Section 5.3

9. $7(-7)$

10. $(-9)(-11)$

11. $\dfrac{-27}{-3}$

12. $\dfrac{14}{-42}$

Section 5.4

13. $5a + 6a - 7$

14. $7xy + 4x - 8xy$

15. $-10x - 4 + 6x - 10$

16. $-5x^2 + 7x + 5x^2$

Section 5.5

17. $6(2x + 7y)$

18. $-4(3x - 6)$

19. $-2(x^2 + 6x - 4)$

20. $-(-x^2 + 3x - 7)$

Equations

6.0   Pretest for Equations

Solve the following problems. After taking the test, see "Step-by-Step Solutions" for the answers (pages 276 to 277). Then, see "6.1 Solving Equations by Adding and Subtracting," "6.2 Solving Equations by Multiplying and Dividing," "6.3 Solving Two-Step Equations," and "6.4 Solving Equations When a Variable Occurs Multiple Times" for skill explanations.

Section 6.1

1. $x - 21 = -22$

2. $-18 = x + 37$

Section 6.2

3. $-12x = -60$

4. $\dfrac{-5x}{11} = 35$

Section 6.3

5. $-64 = 6x + 14$

6. $53 - \dfrac{5}{8}x = -102$

Section 6.4

7. $-12n + 84 = -8n$

8. $3(x - 6) = 2(x + 3)$

9. $4x - 4 + 5x - 3 = -4x - 46$

10. $4(a - 3) = 3 - (a + 5)$

Solving Equations with Addition and Subtraction

In this section, we will review:
- finding the unknown
- inverse operations
- solving to find the value of a variable
- general guidelines for equations

Finding the Unknown

In algebra, equations are used to find an **unknown value** that is represented by a variable (letter). Although any letter of the alphabet can represent the unknown value, the most commonly used letter is x. All equations have an equal sign (=). For example, $x + 5 = 9$ is an equation.

The goal in solving an equation is to find the value of x that makes the equation true.

An equation has two sides, one to the left of the equal sign and one to the right of the sign. Think of the two sides as being on a balance scale. Whatever you do to one side, you must do to the other to keep the scale balanced, or the sides equal (=).

Addition, subtraction, multiplication, and division are the operations used to solve equations.

Inverse Operations

When you move letters and numbers from one side of an equation to the other, you perform inverse operations to keep the equation balanced. **Inverse operations** (opposite) undo each other in equations. Addition and subtraction are inverse operations. Multiplication and division are inverse operations.

Working with a Variable

Before solving an equation, determine if the variable is to the left of the equal sign. If the variable is to the right of the sign, flip the equation. That is, rewrite the equation so that the variable is on the left. For example:

$$9 = x + 3 \quad \text{FLIP: } x + 3 = 9$$

General Guidelines for Equations

When working on any equation, keep these points in mind:

- Work neatly keeping variables, numbers, and the = sign in columns to avoid confusion.
- Apply the rules for positive and negative numbers.
- If the answer is a fraction, reduce it if necessary. If the answer is an improper fraction, reduce it if needed but do not change it to a mixed number.

Tip: Keep things equal—the same number can be added to or subtracted from both sides of an equation without changing the value of the equation.

To solve an equation by adding or subtracting, follow these steps:

1. Make certain that the variable is on the left side of the equal sign. If it is not, flip the equation.
2. Determine the inverse operation. Then either add the same number to both sides of the equation or subtract the same number from both sides of the equation.
3. Add the columns vertically, beginning on the left side of the equation.
4. Simplify the answer if needed.

Example 1: $x + 4 = 6$

STEP 1. Observe that the variable, x, is on the left side of the equal sign.

$$x + 4 = 6$$

STEP 2. Subtract 4 from both sides of the equation since subtraction is the inverse of addition.

$$- 4 = -4$$

STEP 3. Add the columns vertically, beginning with the far left column. First, bring down the x. Next, add: $+4 + (-4) = 0$. Then add: $6 + (-4) = 2$.

$$x + 0 = 2$$

STEP 4. Simplify the answer.

$$x = 2$$

The answer is $x = 2$.

Your work should look like this on paper.

$$x + 4 = 6$$
$$-4 = -4$$
$$x + 0 = 2$$
$$x = 2$$

To check the answer, substitute 2 for x in the original equation.

$$x + 4 = 6$$
$$2 + 4 = 6$$
$$6 = 6 \checkmark \text{ The answer checks.}$$

Example 2: $-7 = x - 3$

STEP 1. Flip the equation since the variable, x, is not on the left side of the equal sign.

$$x - 3 = -7$$

STEP 2. Add 3 to both sides of the equation since addition is the inverse of subtraction.

$$+3 = +3$$

STEP 3. Add the columns vertically, beginning with the far left column. First, bring down the x. Next, add: $(-3) + (3) = 0$. Then add: $(-7) + 3 = -4$.

$$x + 0 = -4$$

STEP 4. Simplify the answer.

$$x = -4$$

The answer is $x = -4$.

Your work should look like this on paper.

$$-7 = x - 3$$
$$x - 3 = -7$$
$$+3 = +3$$
$$x = -4$$

To check the answer, substitute –4 for x in the original equation.

$$-7 = x - 3$$
$$-7 = -4 - 3$$
$$-7 = -7$$ ✔ The answer checks.

6.1 Practice Solving Equations by Adding and Subtracting

Solve the following equations and check your answers. For the answers, see "Step-by-Step Solutions" (pages 277 to 278).

1. $x + 9 = 10$

2. $x - 3 = -8$

3. $y - 6 = 4$

4. $x + 5 = -10$

5. $4 = b + 7$

6. $y + 11 = -6$

7. $x - 7 = -5$

8. $s - 4 = 10$

9. $-7 = x + 5$

10. $y + 15 = 10$

11. $x + 4.1 = 9.2$

12. $a - 3 = 12$

13. $x - 16 = 0$

14. $x + 7.5 = -3.4$

15. $x - 12 = -15$

16. $51 = h - 22$

17. $x - 3 = -1$

18. $x + 5 = -14$

19. $-3 = k - 8$

20. $x - 5 = 13$

Solving Equations by Multiplying and Dividing
In this section, we will review:
- equations that contain multiplication and division
- solving for positive x

Equations that Contain Multiplication and Division

Equations that contain multiplication and division are also solved using inverse operations.

Tip: Keep things equal—both sides of an equation can be multiplied or divided by the same number (except zero) without changing the value of the equation.

To solve equations containing multiplication and division, follow these steps:

1. Flip the equation if the variable is not on the left side of the equal sign.
2. Determine the inverse operation. Then perform either multiplication or division.
3. Use a horizontal fraction bar when division is needed in the equation.
4. Multiply both sides of the equation by a reciprocal if the coefficient of a variable is a fraction, like $\frac{3}{4}x$. Remember, fraction rules state that you cannot divide by a fraction. Instead, you multiply by the reciprocal.
5. Always multiply or divide by the coefficient of the variable along with its sign (positive or negative) to result in a positive x.
6. After solving an equation, **you may end with −x = some number.** If this happens, additional steps are necessary to find **positive x.** Remember that **−x** has a coefficient of **−1** and means **−1x**.

Solving for Positive x

You can solve for positive x in two ways: You can either multiply both sides of the equation by −1 or divide both sides by −1 to get the desired coefficient of x, which is positive 1. The equation is not solved until you reach the step, positive x = some number. For example:

Multiplying both sides by −1

$$-x = -5$$

$$(-1)(-x) = (-5)(-1)$$

$$x = 5$$

Dividing both sides by −1

$$-x = -5$$

$$\frac{-x}{-1} = \frac{-5}{-1}$$

$$x = 5$$

Tip: *Important!* The step-by-step solutions in this book use dividing both sides by −1 to solve for positive x.

Example 1: 4x = 20

STEP 1. Observe that the variable x is on the left side of the equal sign.

$$4x = 20$$

STEP 2. Divide both sides of the equation by 4 since division is the inverse of multiplication. Indicate division by using the fraction bar.

$$\frac{4x}{4} = \frac{20}{4}$$

STEP 3. Reduce fractions, if needed.

$$\frac{\overset{1}{\cancel{4}}x}{\underset{1}{\cancel{4}}} = \frac{\overset{5}{\cancel{20}}}{\underset{1}{\cancel{4}}}$$

STEP 4. Simplify the answer.

$$x = 5$$

The answer is x = 5.

Your work should look like this on paper.

$$4x = 20$$

$$\frac{\overset{1}{\cancel{4}}x}{\underset{1}{\cancel{4}}} = \frac{\overset{5}{\cancel{20}}}{\underset{1}{\cancel{4}}}$$

$$x = 5$$

To check the answer, substitute 5 for x in the original equation.

$$4x = 20$$
$$4(5) = 20$$
$$20 = 20 \quad ✔ \text{ The answer checks.}$$

Example 2: $4 = \dfrac{x}{8}$

STEP 1. Flip the equation since the variable, x, is not on the left side of the equal sign. This equation is read x divided by 8 equals 4.

$$\dfrac{x}{8} = 4$$

STEP 2. Multiply both sides of the equation by 8 since multiplication is the inverse of division.

$$8 \cdot \dfrac{x}{8} = 4 \cdot 8$$

STEP 3. Recall that x means 1x. Therefore, $\dfrac{x}{8}$ means the same as $\dfrac{1x}{8}$. Write all terms of the equation in fraction form.

$$\dfrac{8}{1} \cdot \dfrac{x}{8} = \dfrac{4}{1} \cdot \dfrac{8}{1}$$

STEP 4. Cross cancel.

$$\dfrac{\cancel{8}^{1}}{1} \cdot \dfrac{x}{\cancel{8}_{1}} = \dfrac{4}{1} \cdot \dfrac{8}{1}$$

STEP 5. Multiply the numerators and denominators, then simplify.

$$x = 32$$

The answer is x = 32.

Your work should look like this on paper.

$$4 = \dfrac{x}{8}$$

$$\dfrac{x}{8} = 4$$

$$\overset{1}{\cancel{8}} \cdot \dfrac{x}{\underset{1}{\cancel{8}}} = 4 \cdot 8$$

$$x = 32$$

To check the answer, substitute 32 for x in the original equation.

$$4 = \dfrac{x}{8}$$

$$4 = \dfrac{32}{8}$$

$$4 = 4 \quad ✔ \text{ The answer checks.}$$

Example 3: $-\dfrac{2}{3}x = 12$

STEP 1. Observe that the variable x is on the left side of the equal sign.

$$-\dfrac{2}{3}x = 12$$

STEP 2. Multiply both sides of the equation by $-\dfrac{3}{2}$. Since you cannot divide by a fraction, multiply by the reciprocal of $-\dfrac{2}{3}$.

$$\left(-\dfrac{3}{2}\right)\left(-\dfrac{2}{3}\right)x = 12\left(-\dfrac{3}{2}\right)$$

STEP 3. Write all numbers in the equation in fraction form.

$$\left(-\dfrac{3}{2}\right)\left(-\dfrac{2}{3}\right)x = \left(\dfrac{12}{1}\right)\left(-\dfrac{3}{2}\right)$$

STEP 4. Cross cancel.

$$\left(-\dfrac{\overset{1}{\cancel{3}}}{\underset{1}{\cancel{2}}}\right)\left(-\dfrac{\overset{1}{\cancel{2}}}{\underset{1}{\cancel{3}}}\right)x = \left(\dfrac{\overset{6}{\cancel{12}}}{1}\right)\left(-\dfrac{3}{\underset{1}{\cancel{2}}}\right)$$

STEP 5. Multiply the numerators and denominators, then simplify.

$$x = -18$$

The answer is $x = -18$.

Your work should look like this on paper.

$$-\frac{2}{3}x = 12$$

$$\left(-\frac{3}{2}\right)\left(-\frac{2}{3}\right)x = \left(\frac{12}{1}\right)\left(-\frac{3}{2}\right)$$

$$x = -18$$

To check the answer, substitute −18 for x in the original equation.

$$-\frac{2}{3}x = 12$$

$$\left(-\frac{2}{3}\right)(-18) = 12$$

$$\left(-\frac{2}{3}\right)\left(-\frac{18}{1}\right) = 12$$

$$12 = 12 \quad ✔ \text{ The answer checks.}$$

6.2 Practice Solving Equations by Multiplying and Dividing

Solve the following equations and check your answers. For the answers, see "Step-by-Step Solutions" (pages 278 to 279).

1. $5x = 90$

2. $\dfrac{-m}{5} = 12$

3. $\dfrac{x}{10} = 25$

4. $86 = 2v$

5. $\dfrac{k}{-2} = 37$

6. $-12p = -132$

7. $\dfrac{-h}{7} = 20$

8. $95 = -5y$

9. $3m = -384$

10. $-21r = 672$

11. $\dfrac{x}{100} = 7$

12. $-3 = \dfrac{a}{45}$

13. $-18p = -306$

14. $\dfrac{b}{-9} = -7$

15. $5x = -200$

16. $-84 = \dfrac{2x}{7}$

17. $\dfrac{-x}{4} = -4$

18. $-4x = 120$

19. $\dfrac{-3x}{8} = 24$

20. $-12y = -156$

Solving Two-Step Equations
In this section, we will review:
- equations requiring two operations to solve
- placement of the negative sign in fractions

Two-Step Equations

Two-step equations contain both addition or subtraction and multiplication or division. To solve such equations, follow the order of operations: add or subtract before multiplying or dividing. As a result, you will have these two steps:

1. Start by adding or subtracting.
2. Solve by multiplying or dividing.

Example 1: $3x + 7 = 22$

STEP 1. Subtract 7 from both sides of the equation since subtraction is the inverse of addition.

$$3x + 7 = 22$$
$$-7 = -7$$

STEP 2. Add the columns.

$$3x = 15$$

STEP 3. Divide both sides of the equation by 3 since division is the inverse of multiplication.

$$\frac{3x}{3} = \frac{15}{3}$$

STEP 4. Reduce the fractions on both sides of the equation.

$$\frac{\cancel{3}^{1}x}{\cancel{3}_{1}} = \frac{\cancel{15}^{5}}{\cancel{3}_{1}}$$

STEP 5. Simplify both sides of the equation.

$$x = 5$$

The answer is $x = 5$.

Your work should look like this on paper

$$3x + 7 = 22$$
$$ -7 = -7$$
$$\frac{3x}{3} = \frac{15}{3}$$
$$x = 5$$

To check the answer, substitute 5 for x in the original equation.

$$3(5) + 7 = 22$$
$$15 + 7 = 22$$
$$22 = 22 \quad ✔ \text{ The answer checks.}$$

Example 2: $26 = -5x - 4$

STEP 1. Flip the equation since the variable, x, is not on the left side of the equal sign.

$$-5x - 4 = 26$$

STEP 2. Add 4 to both sides of the equation since addition is the inverse of subtraction.

$$+ 4 = +4$$

STEP 3. Add the columns.

$$-5x = 30$$

STEP 4. Divide both sides of the equation by −5 since division is the inverse of multiplication.

$$\frac{-5x}{-5} = \frac{30}{-5}$$

STEP 5. Reduce the fractions on both sides of the equation.

$$\frac{-5x}{-5} = \frac{30}{-5}$$

STEP 6. Simplify both sides of the equation.

$$x = -6$$

The answer is $x = -6$.

Your work should look like this on paper.

$$26 = -5x - 4$$
$$-5x - 4 = 26$$
$$+4 = +4$$

$$\frac{-5x}{-5} = \frac{30}{-5}$$

$$x = -6$$

To check the answer, substitute –6 for x in the original equation.

$$26 = -5x - 4$$
$$26 = (-5)(-6) - 4$$
$$26 = 30 - 4$$
$$26 = 26 \quad \checkmark \text{ The answer checks.}$$

Example 3: $\dfrac{-x}{4} + 6 = -14$

STEP 1. Subtract 6 from both sides of the equation since subtraction is the inverse of addition.

$$\frac{-x}{4} + 6 = -14$$
$$- 6 = - 6$$

STEP 2. Add the columns.

$$\frac{-x}{4} = -20$$

STEP 3. Multiply both sides of the equation by 4 since multiplication is the inverse of division.

$$4 \cdot \frac{-x}{4} = -20 \cdot 4$$

STEP 4. Write all terms of the equation in fraction form and cross cancel.

$$\frac{4}{1} \cdot \frac{-x}{4} = \frac{-20}{1} \cdot \frac{4}{1}$$

STEP 5. Multiply the numerators and denominators, then simplify.

$$-x = -80$$

STEP 6. Notice that you have not solved for **positive** x. Divide both sides by -1 to solve for **positive** x.

$$\frac{-x}{-1} = \frac{-80}{-1}$$

STEP 7. Simplify the fractions. Now you have solved for **positive** x.

x = 80

The answer is x = 80.

Your work should look like this on paper.

$$\frac{-x}{4} + 6 = -14$$
$$-6 = -6$$
$$\overline{}$$
$$\frac{-x}{4} = -20$$

$$\overset{1}{4} \cdot \frac{-x}{4_1} = -20 \cdot 4$$

$$\frac{-x}{-1} = \frac{-80}{-1}$$
$$x = 80$$

To check the answer, substitute 80 for x in the original equation.

$$\left(\frac{-80}{4}\right) + 6 = -14$$
$$(-20) + 6 = -14$$
$$-14 = -14 \quad \checkmark \text{ The answer checks.}$$

Placement of the Negative Sign in Fractions

Fractions that contain a negative sign may appear in different ways. The fractions $\frac{-2}{3}$, $\frac{2}{-3}$, and $-\frac{2}{3}$ all have the same meaning. A negative fraction in best mathematical form is written with the negative sign in front of the fraction, $-\frac{2}{3}$.

Example 4: $\dfrac{-2x}{7} + 24 = 29$

STEP 1. Subtract 24 from both sides of the equation since subtraction is the inverse of addition.

$$\dfrac{-2x}{7} + 24 = 29$$
$$\underline{ -24 = -24}$$

STEP 2. Add the columns.

$$\dfrac{-2x}{7} = 5$$

STEP 3. Multiply both sides of the equation by $-\dfrac{7}{2}$. Since you cannot divide by a fraction, multiply by the reciprocal of $-\dfrac{2}{7}$.

$$\left(\dfrac{-7}{2}\right)\left(\dfrac{-2x}{7}\right) = 5\left(\dfrac{-7}{2}\right)$$

STEP 4. Write all terms of the equation in fraction form.

$$\left(\dfrac{-7}{2}\right)\left(\dfrac{-2x}{7}\right) = \dfrac{5}{1}\left(\dfrac{-7}{2}\right)$$

STEP 5. Cross cancel.

$$\left(\dfrac{-\overset{1}{7}}{\underset{1}{2}}\right)\left(\dfrac{-\overset{1}{2}x}{\underset{1}{7}}\right) = \dfrac{5}{1}\left(\dfrac{-7}{2}\right)$$

STEP 6. Multiply the numerators and denominators, then simplify. Leave the answer in reduced form as an improper fraction.

$$x = -\dfrac{35}{2}$$

The answer is $x = -\dfrac{35}{2}$.

Your work should look like this on paper.

$$\frac{-2x}{7} + \cancel{24} = 29$$

$$\cancel{-24} = -24$$

$$\frac{-2x}{7} = 5$$

$$\left(\frac{-\cancel{7}^1}{\cancel{2}_1}\right)\left(\frac{-\cancel{2}x}{\cancel{7}}\right)^1 = \frac{5}{1}\left(\frac{-7}{2}\right)$$

$$x = -\frac{35}{2}$$

To check the answer, substitute $-\frac{35}{2}$ for x in the original equation.

$$\frac{-2}{7}x + 24 = 29$$

$$\left(\frac{-\cancel{2}}{\cancel{7}}\right)\left(-\frac{\cancel{35}^5}{\cancel{2}}\right) + 24 = 29$$

$$5 + 24 = 29$$

$$29 = 29 \qquad ✔ \text{The answer checks.}$$

6.3 Practice Solving Two-Step Equations

Solve the following two-step equations and check your answer. For the answers, see "Step-by-Step Solutions" (pages 280 to 281).

1. $4d + 5 = 85$

2. $2r - 7 = 1$

3. $-8 = -2b + 4$

4. $\frac{1}{6}x + 9 = 12$

5. $\frac{b}{7} + 7 = 19$

6. $\frac{x}{4} - 12 = 9$

7. $-t - 8 = -25$

8. $-7m + 1.2 = 4$

9. $9 = \frac{n}{4} - 3$

10. $\frac{y}{3} + 6 = -45$

11. $\frac{-p}{3} + 13 = -4$

12. $-y + 0.6 = 1.8$

13. $\frac{2x}{5} + 17 = 9$

14. $2 = 14 - \frac{3}{4}x$

15. $-5x - 12 = -2$

16. $-2x + 3 = 2$

17. $67 - \frac{3}{4}x = 85$

18. $\frac{2}{3}x - 9 = 11$

19. $2 = -3x - 10$

20. $\frac{5}{7}x - 13 = 82$

Solving Equations When a Variable Occurs Multiple Times
In this section, we will review:
- dealing with more than one variable
- collecting like terms in equations

Dealing with More Than One Variable

All of the equations up to this point have contained only one variable. However, a variable may occur two or more times in an equation. It may be repeated on the same side of the equation or appear on both sides of the equation.

The following equations have the same variable on both sides:

$$-x - 4 = -13x$$
$$4y + 3 = 7(y + 1)$$
$$3(a + 22) = 3(4a + 10)$$

The following equations have the same variable repeated on one or both sides of the equation:

$$6 + x - 2x + 3x - 4x = 3x + 4 - 7x$$
$$7y + 2(2y - 1) = -(4y + 5)$$

Collecting Like Terms in Equations

If an equation has more than one variable term or number on one or both sides of the equal sign, you must collect like terms before moving letters and numbers from one side of the equal sign to the other. For example:

$x + 3x + 4 = -x + 5 - 8$ (before like terms have been collected).
$4x + 4 = -x - 3$ (after like terms have been collected).

After like terms have been collected, move letters to the left side of the equation. Then move numbers to the right side of the equation, so the answer is in best form.

These are the steps for solving an equation that contains more than one variable.

1. Clear parentheses on one or both sides by using the distributive property. (See Section 5.5, The Distributive Property, page 132.)
2. Collect like terms on each side of the equation.
3. Move letters to the left side of the equation.
4. Add or subtract.

5. Move numbers to the right side of the equation.
6. Add or subtract.
7. Multiply or divide as needed.
8. Make certain you have solved for **positive** x.

Tip: You may not need all eight steps to solve every equation; however, you should consider all the steps. If a step is not needed, proceed to the next step.

Example 1: $3n - 5 = -2n$

STEP 1. Observe that there are no parentheses to clear.

$$3n - 5 = -2n$$

STEP 2. Notice that there are no like terms to collect.

STEP 3. Move $-2n$ to the left side of the equation by adding 2n to both sides.

$$+2n \qquad = +2n$$

STEP 4. Add the columns. Note: $-2n + 2n = 0$. Be sure to write the 0 in that column.

$$5n - 5 = \quad 0$$

STEP 5. Move the number 5 to the right side of the equation by adding 5 to both sides.

$$+ 5 = +5$$

STEP 6. Add the columns.

$$5n = 5$$

STEP 7. Divide both sides of the equation by 5.

$$\frac{5n}{5} = \frac{5}{5}$$

STEP 8. Reduce the fractions and be sure you have solved for **positive** n.

$$\frac{\overset{1}{\cancel{5}}n}{\cancel{5}_1} = \frac{\overset{1}{\cancel{5}}}{\cancel{5}_1}$$

The answer is $n = 1$.

$$n = 1$$

Your work should look like this on paper.

$$3n - 5 = \cancel{-2n}$$
$$+2n \quad\;\; = \cancel{+2n}$$
$$\overline{5n \cancel{-5} = \quad 0}$$
$$\quad \cancel{+5} = +5$$
$$\overline{\qquad\qquad\qquad}$$
$$\frac{\overset{1}{\cancel{5}}n}{\underset{1}{\cancel{5}}} = \frac{\overset{1}{\cancel{5}}}{\underset{1}{\cancel{5}}}$$
$$n = 1$$

To check the answer, substitute 1 for x in the original equation.

$$3n - 5 = -2n$$
$$3(1) - 5 = -2(1)$$
$$3 - 5 = -2$$
$$-2 = -2 \qquad \checkmark \text{ The answer checks.}$$

Example 2: $4x - 9 = 7x + 12$

STEP 1. Observe that there are no parentheses to clear.

$$4x - 9 = 7x + 12$$

STEP 2. Notice that there are no like terms to collect.

STEP 3. Move –7x to the left side of the equation by subtracting 7x from both sides.

$$-7x \qquad = -7x$$
$$\overline{\qquad\qquad\qquad}$$

STEP 4. Add the columns.

$$-3x - 9 = 12$$

STEP 5. Move the number –9 to the right side of the equation by adding 9 to both sides.

$$+9 = +9$$
$$\overline{\qquad\qquad\qquad}$$

STEP 6. Add the columns.

$$-3x = 21$$

STEP 7. Divide both sides of the equation by –3.

$$\frac{-3x}{-3} = \frac{21}{-3}$$

STEP 8. Reduce the fractions and be sure you have solved for **positive** x.

$$\frac{\overset{1}{\cancel{-3}}x}{\underset{1}{\cancel{-3}}} = \frac{\cancel{21}^{7}}{\underset{1}{\cancel{-3}}}$$

The answer is x = –7.

$$x = -7$$

Your work should look like this on paper.

$$4x - 9 = \cancel{7x} + 12$$
$$\underline{-7x \quad\quad = \cancel{-7x}}$$
$$-3x - 9 = 12$$
$$\underline{\quad\quad +9 = +9}$$
$$\frac{\overset{1}{\cancel{-3}}x}{\underset{1}{\cancel{-3}}} = \frac{\cancel{21}^{7}}{\underset{1}{\cancel{-3}}}$$
$$x = -7$$

To check the answer, substitute –7 for x in the original equation.

$$4x - 9 = 7x + 12$$
$$4(-7) - 9 = 7(-7) + 12$$
$$-28 - 9 = -49 + 12$$
$$-37 = -37 \qquad ✔ \text{The answer checks.}$$

Example 3: $-6(2x + 5) = 2(3x + 12)$

STEP 1. Use the distributive property to clear the parentheses on both sides.

$$-6(2x + 5) = 2(3x + 12)$$
$$-12x - 30 = 6x + 24$$

STEP 2. Notice that there are no like terms to collect.

STEP 3. Move 6x to the left side of the equation by subtracting 6x from both sides.

$$- 6x \qquad = - 6x$$

STEP 4. Add the columns.

$$-18x - 30 = 24$$

STEP 5. Move the number -30 to the right side of the equation by adding 30 to both sides.

$$+ 30 = +30$$

STEP 6. Add the columns.

$$-18x = 54$$

STEP 7. Divide both sides of the equation by 18.

$$\frac{-18x}{18} = \frac{54}{18}$$

STEP 8. Reduce the fractions.

$$\frac{\overset{1}{\cancel{-18}}x}{\underset{1}{\cancel{18}}} = \frac{\overset{3}{\cancel{54}}}{\underset{1}{\cancel{18}}}$$

STEP 9. Notice that you have not solved for **positive** x.

$$-x = 3$$

STEP 10. Divide both sides by −1 to solve for **positive** x.

$$\frac{-x}{-1} = \frac{3}{-1}$$

STEP 11. Simplify the fractions. Now you have solved for **positive** x.

$$x = -3$$

The answer is x = −3.

Your work should look like this on paper.

$$-6(2x + 5) = 2(3x + 12)$$

$$-12x - 30 = \cancel{6x} + 24$$

$$\underline{-6x \qquad = \cancel{-6x}}$$

$$-18x - \cancel{30} = 24$$

$$\underline{+\cancel{30} = + 30}$$

$$\frac{-\overset{1}{\cancel{18}}x}{\underset{1}{\cancel{18}}} = \frac{\overset{3}{\cancel{54}}}{\underset{1}{\cancel{18}}}$$

$$\frac{-x}{-1} = \frac{3}{-1}$$

$$x = -3$$

To check the answer, substitute -3 for x in the original equation.

$$-6(2x + 5) = 2(3x + 12)$$

$$-6[2(-3) + 5] = 2[3(-3) + 12]$$

$$-6[-6 + 5] = 2[-9 + 12]$$

$$-6[-1] = 2[3]$$

$$6 = 6 \quad ✔ \text{ The answer checks.}$$

Tip: Here is why Example 3, Step 9 is $-x = 3$: You can solve Step 9 in two ways—

Choice 1	Choice 2

$$\frac{-\overset{1}{\cancel{18}}x}{\underset{1}{\cancel{18}}} = \frac{\overset{3}{\cancel{54}}}{\underset{1}{\cancel{18}}} \qquad\qquad \frac{-\overset{1}{\cancel{18}}x}{\underset{1}{\cancel{-18}}} = \frac{\overset{3}{\cancel{54}}}{\underset{1}{\cancel{-18}}}$$

$$-x = 3 \qquad\qquad\qquad x = -3$$

$$\frac{-x}{-1} = \frac{3}{-1}$$

$$x = -3$$

In Choice 1, $\dfrac{-\cancel{18}x}{\cancel{18}} = -x$. Two additional steps are needed to solve for

positive x to complete the problem.

To eliminate extra steps and solve the equation for positive x, follow

this process. Recall the rules: $\dfrac{+}{+}$ or $\dfrac{-}{-} = +$. In the final division step of

an equation, if the coefficient of x is positive, then divide by a positive number. If it is negative, then divide by a negative number as shown in Choice 2.

Example 4: $3(3x + 4) - 7 = 3x - 5x + 27$

STEP 1. Clear the parentheses on one or both sides by using the distributive property.

$$3(3x + 4) - 7 = 3x - 5x + 27$$
$$9x + 12 - 7 = 3x - 5x + 27$$

STEP 2. Collect like terms on each side of the equation.

$$9x + 5 = -2x + 27$$

STEP 3. Move –2x to the left side of the equation by adding 2x to both sides.

$$+2x \qquad = +2x$$

STEP 4. Add the columns.

$$11x + 5 = 27$$

STEP 5. Move the number 5 to the right side of the equation by subtracting 5 from both sides.

$$-5 = -5$$

STEP 6. Add the columns.

$$11x = 22$$

STEP 7. Divide both sides by 11.

$$\frac{11x}{11} = \frac{22}{11}$$

STEP 8. Reduce the fractions. Be sure
you have solved for **positive** x.

$$\frac{\overset{1}{\cancel{11}}x}{\underset{1}{\cancel{11}}} = \frac{\overset{2}{\cancel{22}}}{\underset{1}{\cancel{11}}}$$

The answer is x = 2.

$$x = 2$$

Your work should look like this on paper.

$$3(\overparen{3x + 4}) -7 = 3x - 5x + 27$$
$$9x + 12 - 7 = 3x - 5x + 27$$
$$9x + 5 = -\cancel{2}x + 27$$
$$\underline{+2x \qquad = +\cancel{2}x}$$
$$11x + \cancel{5} = 27$$
$$\underline{-\cancel{5} = -5}$$
$$\frac{\overset{1}{\cancel{11}}x}{\underset{1}{\cancel{11}}} = \frac{\overset{2}{\cancel{22}}}{\underset{1}{\cancel{11}}}$$
$$x = 2$$

To check the answer, substitute 2 for x in the
original equation.

$$3(3x + 4) - 7 = 3x - 5x + 27$$
$$3[(3 \cdot 2) + 4] - 7 = (3 \cdot 2) - (5 \cdot 2) + 27$$
$$3[6 + 4] - 7 = 6 - 10 + 27$$
$$3[10] - 7 = -4 + 27$$
$$30 - 7 = 23$$
$$23 = 23 \qquad ✔ \text{The answer checks.}$$

6.4 Practice Solving Equations When a Variable Occurs Multiple Times

Solve the following equations. For the answers, see "Step-by-Step Solutions" (pages 282 to 285).

1. $-9x - 72 = 3x$

2. $3x + 3 = x - 5$

3. $2x - 11 = -8x + 109$

4. $6 - 8x = 20x + 20$

5. $-x - 4 = -13x - 100$

6. $3(k + 2) = 12k$

7. $4y + 3 = 7(y + 1)$

8. $2(x + 1) = 3x - 1$

9. $3(a + 22) = 3(4a + 10)$

10. $5(z - 1) = 4(z + 4)$

11. $6(y + 3) = 4(y + 9)$

12. $7x - 6 - 9x = 12x - 48$

13. $3x - x - 5 = x + 8$

14. $4x + 4 - 2x - x = 4x - 5$

15. $6 + x - 2x + 3x - 4x = 3x + 4$

16. $5m - (m + 5) = 11$

17. $y + 2(y - 3) = 4 - 2y$

18. $-2(x - 4) - x = -x - 2$

19. $2m - 3(m + 3) = -13(m + 1)$

20. $7y + 2(2y - 1) = -(4y + 5)$

Solve the following problems. After taking the test, see "Step-by-Step Solutions" for the answers (pages 285 to 287). And, see "6.1 Solving Equations by Adding and Subtracting," "6.2 Solving Equations by Multiplying and Dividing," "6.3 Solving Two-Step Equations," and "6.4 Solving Equations When a Variable Occurs Multiple Times" if the chapter test indicates you need additional practice on any skill.

Section 6.1

1. $x + 4 = 9$

2. $x - 17 = 35$

3. $k + 91 = -22$

4. $-36 = x - 12$

Section 6.2

5. $5r = -35$

6. $-81 = -9x$

7. $\dfrac{x}{8} = -16$

8. $\dfrac{-4}{9} d = -20$

Section 6.3

9. $5y - 4 = 26$

10. $\dfrac{-x}{4} + 6 = -14$

11. $2 = -3c - 10$

12. $8 - \dfrac{1}{5}x = 5$

Section 6.4

13. $9n - 15 = 6n$

14. $4x - 9 = 7x - 12$

15. $6y - 3 = 3(y + 2)$

16. $5m - 2m + 4 = 3m + m - 1$

17. $5(3x + 6) = 3(x + 18)$

18. $-4x - 3 + 2x - 6 = -7x + 6$

19. $x - 5 + 4x = 4(x - 3)$

20. $2(y + 8) - 4 = 8y$

Practice Tests for Basic Math Skills

part II

Practice Test 1
Cumulative Skills Test

This test provides sample problems for each math skill presented in Part I. The test will show you which skills you have mastered as well as help you identify any skills for which you need additional practice.

Solve each problem.

For test answers, see "Step-by-Step Solutions," pages 288-294. To the left of each solution, you will notice two numbers. These numbers indicate the chapter and section—for example, (1.2) means Chapter 1, Section 2—where you can find a detailed explanation for solving similar problems. If your answer is incorrect and you need more practice, you may wish to review the indicated material.

1. $\begin{array}{r} 57{,}942 \\ +78{,}859 \\ \hline \end{array}$

2. $\begin{array}{r} 21{,}300 \\ -17{,}452 \\ \hline \end{array}$

3. $\begin{array}{r} 4{,}706 \\ \times 505 \\ \hline \end{array}$

4. Write the quotient with a remainder.

    $530\overline{)25{,}075}$

5. Write in fraction form.

   39

6. Write as a mixed number.

   $\dfrac{36}{5}$

7. Write as an improper fraction.

   $2\dfrac{3}{5}$

8. Are these fractions equivalent?

   $\dfrac{1}{3} = \dfrac{9}{27}$

9. $4 \times \dfrac{7}{9}$

10. $4\dfrac{3}{5} \times 2\dfrac{1}{2} \times 1\dfrac{5}{23}$

11. $\dfrac{5}{8} \div \dfrac{25}{16}$

12. $\dfrac{3}{7} \div 2$

13. $4\dfrac{4}{5} \div \dfrac{8}{3}$

14. Find the least common denominator for these fractions.

    $\dfrac{3}{7}$ and $\dfrac{1}{4}$

15. Find the least common denominator for these fractions.

    $\dfrac{5}{21}$ and $\dfrac{8}{35}$

16. Find the least common denominator for these fractions.

    $\dfrac{7}{15}$ and $\dfrac{11}{12}$ and $\dfrac{5}{8}$

17. $2\dfrac{3}{5} + \dfrac{1}{3} + 6\dfrac{2}{15}$

18. $\dfrac{53}{88} - \dfrac{19}{44}$

19. $26\dfrac{1}{4} - 5\dfrac{5}{6}$

20. Which digit is in the thousandth's place?

14.6597

21. Write $\dfrac{67}{10,000}$ as a decimal number.

22. Write the decimal number two hundred six ten thousandths.

23. Round 346.785 to the nearest hundredth.

24. Round 87,943 to the nearest ten.

25. 4.23 + 1.5 + 7.2341

26. 23.479 − 0.96

27. 0.171 × 0.238

28. 0.6 ÷ 0.02

29. Round the quotient to the nearest tenth.

$24\overline{)539}$

30. Write 0.25 as a reduced fraction.

31. Write $\dfrac{3}{4}$ as a decimal number.

32. Arrange from least to greatest.
0.2   0.02   0.3   0.33

33. Place <, =, or > in the blank.

0.27 _____ $\dfrac{1}{5}$

34. Arrange from least to greatest.

$\dfrac{3}{5}$ $\dfrac{7}{15}$ $\dfrac{11}{30}$

35. $\dfrac{25}{4} = \dfrac{n}{12}$

36. 40 is what percent of 16?

37. 30% of 90 is what?

38. 50 is 20% of what?

39. $12\dfrac{1}{2}$% of what is 15?

40. $\dfrac{3}{16}$ is what percent of $\dfrac{3}{4}$?

41. Write 12.5% as a fraction.

42. Write $\dfrac{6}{18}$ as a percent.

43. Write 6 : 20 as a percent.

44. $\dfrac{6.5}{20\%}$

45. Write 66% as a decimal.

46. Write 0.456 as a percent.

47. $-17 + (-4)$

48. $25 + (-8)$

49. $-36 + 36$

50. $-18 + 10$

51. $13 - 15$

52. $-8 - 19$

53. $-5 - (-23)$

54. $7 - (-4)$

55. $(-9)(-10)$

56. $4(-17)$

57. $\dfrac{-81}{-9}$

58. $\dfrac{-15}{60}$

59. $7x - 3x + 12x$

60. $5xy^2 - 3xy - xy$

61. $(x^2 - 2) - (3x^2 - 4x + 5)$

62. $7(r + 6)$

63. $-3(x^2 + 7x - 9)$

64. $- (a - 10)$

65. $x + 37 = -26$

66. $x - 71 = 23$

67. $-5x = -80$

68. $\dfrac{2}{5}x = -14$

69. $3x + 7 = 22$

70. $13 - \dfrac{3x}{2} = 37$

71. $3x - 10 = -9x$

72. $2(x + 1) = 3x - 1$

73. $2(y + 3) = 4(y - 6)$

74. $3(x + 3) + 5 = 2x$

75. $13 + 5x - 7 = 3x - 8 - 12x$

Practice Test 2
Combined Skills Test

The Combined Skills Test contains problems that require the use of one or more basic math skills. If you are preparing to take a timed, standardized test, this test provides excellent practice.

Set a timer for 30 minutes (1 minute for each problem), write each problem on your paper and solve. Repeat this process until you are able to complete the test in 30 minutes with the desired accuracy.

Table 11:	Score Results
Number Incorrect	**Score**
0-3	A
4-6	B
7-9	C

For test answers, see "Step-by-Step Solutions," pages 295-298. To the left of each solution, you will notice two numbers. These numbers indicate the chapter and section—for example, (1.2) means Chapter 1, Section 2—where you can find a detailed explanation for solving similar problems. If your answer is incorrect and you need more practice, you may wish to review the indicated material.

1. Write $\dfrac{47}{100,000}$ as a decimal number.

2. Which digit is in the hundredth's place?

1,346.979

3. Write the decimal number sixteen and four hundredths.

4. Round 5,642.0182 to the nearest thousandth.

5. 9.6 + 8.234 + 1.05

6. 403.1 − 15.236

7. 14.56 × 0.2

8. 0.903 ÷ 0.43

9. Reduce to lowest terms.

$$\frac{25}{300}$$

10. Write as a mixed number.

$$\frac{50}{7}$$

11. Are these fractions equivalent?

$$\frac{2}{5} = \frac{8}{25}$$

12. $1\frac{1}{4} + 2\frac{5}{6} + \frac{1}{12}$

13. $37\frac{1}{5} - 9\frac{4}{7}$

14. $1\frac{3}{4} \times 2\frac{2}{3} \times 1\frac{4}{5}$

15. $\frac{5}{9} \div 1\frac{1}{3}$

16. Write 62.5% as a reduced common fraction.

17. Write $\frac{1}{8}$ as a decimal number.

18. Write 650% as a decimal.

19. Write $\frac{49}{7}$ as a percent.

20. Write 4 : 20 as a percent.

21. Write 0.017 as a percent.

22. $\frac{13.4}{40\%}$

23. 16.5% of 72 is what?

24. $33\frac{1}{3}$ % of x is 45?

25. 210 is 35% of what?

26. $\frac{1}{2}$ is what percent of $\frac{4}{5}$?

27. $(x^2 - 5) - (-4x^2 + 5x - 1)$

28. $-2v + 4 = -8$

29. $5m + 8 = 3(m + 4)$

30. $4(x - 9) + 12 = -2(x - 6)$

31. Arrange from least to greatest.
0.57   0.507   0.572   0.5

32. Place <, =, or > in the blank.

0.35 _____ $\frac{3}{8}$

33. Arrange from least to greatest.
$\frac{1}{8}$ $\frac{1}{4}$ $\frac{1}{6}$

Measures Used in Health Care Applications

part III

7.0   Pretest for Household Measures

Solve the following problems. After taking the test, see "Step-by-Step Solutions" for the answers (page 299). Then, see "7.1 Household Measures for Length," "7.2 Household Measures for Weight," and "7.3 Household Measures for Volume" for skill explanations.

Sections 7.1 and 7.2

Convert the following measurements.

1. 40 ounces to pounds

2. 4 feet to inches

3. 3 pints to quarts

4. 15 teaspoons to tablespoons

5. 25 feet to yards

6. 6 tablespoons to fluid ounces

7. 5,000 pounds to tons

8. 17 miles to feet

Section 7.3

9. 3 cups to tablespoons

10. 8 pints to gallons

7.1   **Household Measures for Length**
In this section, we will review:
- converting measurements using unit multipliers
- length conversions

Converting Measurements Using Unit Multipliers

Unit multipliers are helpful for making conversions in any measurement system. They are used in some nursing calculations. A unit multiplier is written in fraction form and has a value of 1 if reduced. What makes these fractions unique is that unit multipliers include units of measure along with numbers. For example:

$$12 \text{ inches} = 1 \text{ foot} \qquad \frac{12 \text{ inches}}{1 \text{ foot}} = 1$$

$\dfrac{12 \text{ inches}}{1 \text{ foot}}$ is a unit multiplier.

Multiplying by a unit multiplier, a carefully chosen form of 1, is the key to converting units. Unit multipliers work because you can multiply any number by 1 and not change its value.

Using a Unit Multiplier

To solve a conversion problem by using a unit multiplier, follow these four steps:

1. Write the number and unit given in fraction form.
2. Find the unit multipliers in the chart that contain both units in the problem.
3. Choose the unit multiplier that has the unit you are solving for in the numerator.
4. Multiply the fraction form in STEP 1 by the chosen unit multiplier. Cross cancel numbers and units. Reduce if necessary. Be sure the answer is written in best mathematical form.

Table 7.1	Unit Multipliers for Length	
Length Conversions	**Unit Multipliers**	
12 inches = 1 foot	$\dfrac{12 \text{ in.}}{1 \text{ ft.}}$ or $\dfrac{1 \text{ ft.}}{12 \text{ in.}}$	
3 feet = 1 yard	$\dfrac{3 \text{ ft.}}{1 \text{ yd.}}$ or $\dfrac{1 \text{ yd.}}{3 \text{ ft.}}$	
5,280 feet = 1 mile	$\dfrac{5{,}280 \text{ ft.}}{1 \text{ mi.}}$ or $\dfrac{1 \text{ mi.}}{5{,}280 \text{ ft.}}$	

Length Conversions

The most common units for household length are the inch, foot, yard, and mile. See Table 7.1 for common conversions and the corresponding unit multipliers. Note that each conversion has two corresponding unit multipliers, which are reciprocals.

Example 1: Convert 6 inches to feet.

STEP 1. Write 6 inches in fraction form.

$$\frac{6 \text{ in.}}{1}$$

STEP 2. Find the unit multipliers in the chart that contain both inches and feet.

$$\frac{12 \text{ in.}}{1 \text{ ft.}} \text{ or } \frac{1 \text{ ft.}}{12 \text{ in.}}$$

STEP 3. Choose the unit multiplier that has the unit you are solving for (feet) in the numerator.

$$\frac{1 \text{ ft.}}{12 \text{ in.}}$$

STEP 4. Multiply the fraction form in STEP 1 by the chosen unit multiplier. Cross cancel numbers and units. Reduce if necessary. Write the answer in best form.

$$\frac{\overset{1}{\cancel{6 \text{ in.}}}}{1} \cdot \frac{1 \text{ ft.}}{\underset{2}{\cancel{12 \text{ in.}}}} = \frac{1 \text{ ft.}}{2} = \frac{1}{2} \text{ foot}$$

The answer is $\dfrac{1}{2}$ foot.

Example 2: Convert 243 feet to yards.

STEP 1. Write 243 feet in fraction form.

$$\frac{243 \text{ ft.}}{1}$$

STEP 2. Find the unit multipliers in the chart that contain both feet and yards.

$$\frac{3 \text{ ft.}}{1 \text{ yd.}} \text{ or } \frac{1 \text{ yd.}}{3 \text{ ft.}}$$

STEP 3. Choose the unit multiplier that has the unit you are solving for (yards) in the numerator.

$$\frac{1 \text{ yd.}}{3 \text{ ft.}}$$

STEP 4. Multiply the fraction form in STEP 1 by the chosen unit multiplier. Cross cancel numbers and units. Reduce if necessary. Write the answer in best form.

$$\frac{\overset{81}{\cancel{243}} \cancel{\text{ ft.}}}{1} \cdot \frac{1 \text{ yd.}}{\underset{1}{\cancel{3}} \cancel{\text{ ft.}}} = \frac{81 \text{ yd.}}{1} = 81 \text{ yards}$$

The answer is 81 yards.

Example 3: Convert 26,400 feet to miles.

STEP 1. Write 26,400 feet in fraction form.

$$\frac{26,400 \text{ ft.}}{1}$$

STEP 2. Find the unit multipliers in the chart that contain both feet and miles.

$$\frac{5,280 \text{ ft.}}{1 \text{ mi.}} \text{ or } \frac{1 \text{ mi.}}{5,280 \text{ ft.}}$$

STEP 3. Choose the unit multiplier that has the unit you are solving for (miles) in the numerator.

$$\frac{1 \text{ mi.}}{5,280 \text{ ft.}}$$

STEP 4. Multiply the fraction form in STEP 1 by the chosen unit multiplier. Cross cancel numbers and units. Reduce if necessary. Write the answer in best form.

$$\overset{5}{\cancel{26,400}} \text{ ft.} \cdot \frac{1 \text{ mi.}}{\underset{1}{\cancel{5,280}} \text{ ft.}} = \frac{5 \text{ mi.}}{1} = 5 \text{ miles}$$

The answer is 5 miles.

7.1 Practice Household Measures for Length Conversions

Convert the following measurements using a unit multiplier. For the answers, see "Step-by-Step Solutions" (pages 300 to 301).

1. 9 feet to inches

2. 72 inches to feet

3. 4 miles to feet

4. 6 feet to yards

5. 9,240 feet to miles

6. 430 feet to yards

7. 120 inches to feet

8. 18 miles to feet

9. 42 feet to inches

10. 33 feet to yards

11. 720 yards to feet

12. 7,920 feet to miles

13. 30 feet to inches

14. 693 feet to yards

15. 30 inches to feet

16. 10 miles to feet

17. 27,720 feet to miles

18. 29 yards to feet

19. 10 feet to yards

20. 1.25 miles to feet

Household Measures for Weight
In this section, we will review:
- using a unit multiplier
- weight conversions

Using a Unit Multiplier

To use a unit multiplier, follow the steps listed in Section 7.1 Household Measures for Length, page 176.

Tip: All types of conversion problems—length, weight, or volume—that require one unit multiplier can be solved by applying the four steps for using a unit multiplier.

Weight Conversions

The most common units for household weight are the ounce, pound, and ton. See Table 7.2 for common conversions and the corresponding unit multipliers. Note that each conversion has two corresponding unit multipliers, which are reciprocals.

Table 7.2	Unit Multipliers for Weight
Weight Conversions	**Unit Multipliers**
16 ounces = 1 pound	$\dfrac{16 \text{ oz.}}{1 \text{ lb.}}$ or $\dfrac{1 \text{ lb.}}{16 \text{ oz.}}$
2,000 pounds = 1 ton	$\dfrac{2{,}000 \text{ lbs.}}{1 \text{ ton}}$ or $\dfrac{1 \text{ ton}}{2{,}000 \text{ lbs.}}$

If the conversion contains a fraction, change it to decimal form before solving. For example:

$$1\frac{1}{2} \textbf{ pounds} = \textbf{1.5 pounds}$$

Example 1: Convert 72 ounces to pounds.

STEP 1. Write 72 ounces in fraction form.

$$\frac{72 \text{ oz.}}{1}$$

STEP 2. Find the unit multipliers in the chart that contain both ounces and pounds.

$$\frac{16 \text{ oz.}}{1 \text{ lb.}} \quad \text{or} \quad \frac{1 \text{ lb.}}{16 \text{ oz.}}$$

STEP 3. Choose the unit multiplier that has the unit you are solving for (pounds) in the numerator.

$$\frac{1 \text{ lb.}}{16 \text{ oz.}}$$

STEP 4. Multiply the fraction form in STEP 1 by the chosen unit multiplier. Cross cancel numbers and units. Reduce if necessary. Write the answer in best form.

$$\frac{\overset{9}{\cancel{72}} \text{ oz.}}{1} \cdot \frac{1 \text{ lb.}}{\underset{2}{\cancel{16}} \text{ oz.}} = \frac{9}{2} \text{ lbs.} = 4\frac{1}{2} \text{ pounds}$$

The answer is 4½ pounds.

Example 2: Convert 6,800 pounds to tons.

STEP 1. Write 6,800 pounds in fraction form.

$$\frac{6,800 \text{ lb.}}{1}$$

STEP 2. Find the unit multipliers in the chart that contain both pounds and tons.

$$\frac{2,000 \text{ lb.}}{1 \text{ ton}} \quad \text{or} \quad \frac{1 \text{ ton}}{2,000 \text{ lb.}}$$

STEP 3. Choose the unit multiplier that has the unit you are solving for (tons) in the numerator.

$$\frac{1 \text{ ton}}{2,000 \text{ lb.}}$$

STEP 4. Multiply the fraction form in STEP 1 by the chosen unit multiplier. Cross cancel numbers and units. Reduce if necessary. Write the answer in best form.

$$\frac{6{,}800 \text{ lb.}}{1} \cdot \frac{1 \text{ ton}}{2{,}000 \text{ lb.}} = \frac{17 \text{ tons}}{5} = 3\frac{2}{5} \text{ tons}$$

The answer is $3\frac{2}{5}$ tons.

Example 3: Convert $2\frac{3}{4}$ pounds to ounces.

STEP 1. Change $2\frac{3}{4}$ to a decimal number.

Write 2.75 pounds in fraction form.

$$\frac{2.75 \text{ lb.}}{1}$$

STEP 2. Find the unit multipliers in the chart that contain both pounds and ounces.

$$\frac{16 \text{ oz.}}{1 \text{ lb.}} \text{ or } \frac{1 \text{ lb.}}{16 \text{ oz.}}$$

STEP 3. Choose the unit multiplier that has the unit you are solving for (ounces) in the numerator.

$$\frac{16 \text{ oz.}}{1 \text{ lb.}}$$

STEP 4. Multiply the fraction form in STEP 1 by the chosen unit multiplier. Cross cancel numbers and units. Reduce if necessary. Write the answer in best form.

$$\frac{2.75 \text{ lb.}}{1} \cdot \frac{16 \text{ oz.}}{1 \text{ lb.}} = 44 \text{ ounces}$$

The answer is 44 ounces.

7.2 Practice Weight Conversions

Convert the following measurements using a unit multiplier. For the answers, see "Step-by-Step Solutions" (pages 301 to 303).

1. 32 ounces to pounds

2. 3 pounds to ounces

3. 2.5 tons to pounds

4. 2,500 pounds to tons

5. $5\frac{1}{4}$ pounds to ounces

6. $\frac{3}{4}$ ton to pounds

7. 12 ounces to pounds

8. 3,600 pounds to tons

9. 68 ounces to pounds

10. $1\frac{1}{4}$ pounds to ounces

11. 4 tons to pounds

12. 20,000 pounds to tons

13. 144 ounces to pounds

14. 15,000 pounds to tons

15. 16 ounces to pounds

16. $1\frac{1}{2}$ tons to pounds

17. 112 ounces to pounds

18. 1,000 pounds to tons

19. 16 tons to pounds

20. 5.5 pounds to ounces

Household Measures for Volume
In this section, we will review:
- using two unit multipliers in a conversion
- volume conversions

Using Two Unit Multipliers in a Conversion

For the length and weight conversions shown thus far, only one unit multiplier was required to find the answer. However, some conversions may require more than one unit multiplier. For instance, when no unit multiplier in Table 7.3 shows a direct conversion between units, you will need two or more unit multipliers to link the units to reach the desired unit.

This is the way to think through the conversion process:

- Three terms are multiplied together to find the answer.
- The first term is the number and unit given in the problem written in fraction form.
- The second term is the first unit multiplier. It has the same denominator as the unit given in the first term.
- The third term is the second unit multiplier. It has the units you are trying to find in the numerator.

Volume Conversions

Volume means capacity, or how much something holds. Within the household measurement system, there are many measures and a variety of conversions for volume. See Table 7.3 for the conversions and the corresponding unit multipliers for volume.

Some volume conversions require only one unit multiplier. However, in this section there is no direction conversion shown in the table for the units given in the examples. Therefore, two unit multipliers will be required to complete the conversions.

Table 7.3	Unit Multipliers for Volume	
Measure	**Volume Conversions**	**Unit Multipliers**
tablespoon	1 tablespoon = 3 teaspoons	$\dfrac{1\ T.}{3\ tsp.}$ or $\dfrac{3\ tsp.}{1\ T.}$
fluid ounce	1 fluid ounce = 2 tablespoons	$\dfrac{1\ fl.oz.}{2\ T.}$ or $\dfrac{2\ T.}{1\ fl.oz.}$
cup	1 cup = 8 fluid ounces	$\dfrac{1\ cup}{8\ fl.oz.}$ or $\dfrac{8\ fl.oz.}{1\ cup}$
pint	1 pint = 2 cups	$\dfrac{1\ pt.}{2\ cups}$ or $\dfrac{2\ cups}{1\ pt.}$
quart	1 quart = 2 pints	$\dfrac{1\ qt.}{2\ pt.}$ or $\dfrac{2\ pt.}{1\ qt.}$
gallon	1 gallon = 4 quarts	$\dfrac{1\ gal.}{4\ qt.}$ or $\dfrac{4\ qt.}{1\ gal.}$

Example 1: Convert 12 gallons to pints. Use **2** unit multipliers.

STEP 1. Write a 3-term format to begin. First, write 12 gallons in fraction form. The second term has gallons in the denominator in order to cancel with the numerator in the first term. The third term has the units you are trying to find (pints) in the numerator.

$$\frac{12\ \cancel{gal.}}{1} \cdot \frac{}{\cancel{gal.}} \cdot \frac{pt.}{}$$

STEP 2. Find a unit multiplier in the conversion chart with gallon in the denominator.

$$\frac{4\ qt.}{1\ gal.}$$

STEP 3. Place this unit multiplier in the second term.

$$\frac{12\ \cancel{gal.}}{1} \cdot \frac{4\ qt.}{1\ \cancel{gal.}} \cdot \frac{pt.}{}$$

STEP 4. Observe that the third term must have quart in the denominator to cancel with the quart in the numerator in the second term. Look at the chart and choose the unit multiplier with pint in the numerator and quart in the denominator.

$$\frac{2\ pt.}{1\ qt.}$$

STEP 5. Place this unit multiplier in the third term.

$$\frac{12 \text{ gal.}}{1} \cdot \frac{4 \text{ qt.}}{1 \text{ gal.}} \cdot \frac{2 \text{ pt.}}{1 \text{ qt.}}$$

STEP 6. Cross cancel numbers and units. Multiply remaining numerators and denominators. Reduce if necessary. Write the answer in best form.

$$\frac{12 \text{ gal.}}{1} \cdot \frac{4 \text{ qt.}}{1 \text{ gal.}} \cdot \frac{2 \text{ pt.}}{1 \text{ qt.}} = 96 \text{ pints}$$

The answer is 96 pints.

Example 2: Convert 2 cups to tablespoons. Use **2** unit multipliers.

STEP 1. Write a 3-term format to begin. First, write 2 cups in fraction form. The second term has cup in the denominator in order to cancel with the numerator in the first term. The third term has the units you are trying to find (tablespoons) in the numerator.

$$\frac{2 \text{ cups}}{1} \cdot \frac{}{\text{cup}} \cdot \frac{\text{T.}}{}$$

STEP 2. Find a unit multiplier in the conversion chart with cup in the denominator.

$$\frac{8 \text{ fl.oz.}}{1 \text{ cup}}$$

STEP 3. Place this unit multiplier in the second term.

$$\frac{2 \text{ cups}}{1} \cdot \frac{8 \text{ fl.oz.}}{1 \text{ cup}} \cdot \frac{\text{T.}}{}$$

STEP 4. Observe that the third term must have fluid ounces in the denominator to cancel with the fluid ounces in the numerator in the second term. Look at the chart and choose the unit multiplier with tablespoon in the numerator and fluid ounces in the denominator.

$$\frac{2 \text{ T.}}{1 \text{ fl.oz.}}$$

STEP 5. Place this unit multiplier in the third term.

$$\frac{2 \text{ c}\cancel{\text{ups}}}{1} \cdot \frac{8 \text{ fl.oz.}}{1 \text{ c}\cancel{\text{up}}} \cdot \frac{2 \text{ T.}}{1 \text{ fl.oz.}}$$

STEP 6. Cross cancel numbers and units. Multiply remaining numerators and denominators. Reduce if necessary. Write the answer in best form.

$$\frac{2 \text{ c}\cancel{\text{ups}}}{1} \cdot \frac{8 \text{ f}\cancel{\text{l}}.oz.}{1 \text{ c}\cancel{\text{up}}} \cdot \frac{2 \text{ T.}}{1 \text{ f}\cancel{\text{l}}.oz.} = 32 \text{ tablespoons}$$

The answer is 32 tablespoons.

Example 3: Convert 100 cups to quarts. Use **2** unit multipliers.

STEP 1. Write a 3-term format to begin. First, write 100 cups in fraction form. The second term has cups in the denominator in order to cancel with the numerator in the first term. The third term has the units you are trying to find (quart) in the numerator.

$$\frac{100 \text{ c}\cancel{\text{ups}}}{1} \cdot \frac{}{\text{c}\cancel{\text{ups}}} \cdot \frac{\text{qt.}}{}$$

STEP 2. Find a unit multiplier in the conversion chart with cups in the denominator.

$$\frac{1 \text{ pt.}}{2 \text{ cups}}$$

STEP 3. Place this unit multiplier in the second term.

$$\frac{100 \text{ c}\cancel{\text{ups}}}{1} \cdot \frac{1 \text{ pt.}}{2 \text{ c}\cancel{\text{ups}}} \cdot \frac{\text{qt.}}{}$$

STEP 4. Observe that the third term must have pint in the denominator to cancel with the pint in the numerator in the second term. Look at the chart and choose the unit multiplier with quart in the numerator and pint in the denominator.

$$\frac{1 \text{ qt.}}{2 \text{ pt.}}$$

STEP 5. Place this unit multiplier in the third term.

$$\frac{100 \text{ cups}}{1} \cdot \frac{1 \text{ pt.}}{2 \text{ cups}} \cdot \frac{1 \text{ qt.}}{2 \text{ pt.}}$$

STEP 6. Cross cancel numbers and units. Multiply remaining numerators and denominators. Reduce if necessary. Write the answer in best form.

$$\frac{\overset{25}{\cancel{\underset{50}{100}}} \text{ cups}}{1} \cdot \frac{1 \text{ pt.}}{\underset{1}{\cancel{2}} \text{ cups}} \cdot \frac{1 \text{ qt.}}{\underset{1}{\cancel{2}} \text{ pt.}} = 25 \text{ quarts}$$

The answer is 25 quarts.

7.3 Practice Volume Conversions

Convert the following measurements using one unit multiplier. For the answers, see "Step-by-Step Solutions" (pages 303 to 305).

1. 6 tablespoons to teaspoons

2. 20 quarts to pints

3. 4 gallons to quarts

4. 45 pints to cups

5. 12 fluid ounces to cups

6. 6 gallons to quarts

7. 27 teaspoons to tablespoons

8. 10 cups to pints

9. 22 quarts to gallons

10. 9 teaspoons to tablespoons

*Use **two** unit multipliers from the chart to convert the following measurements.*

11. 26 tablespoons to cups

12. 2 pints to fluid ounces

13. 7 cups to quarts

14. 10 gallons to pints

15. 8 fluid ounces to pints

16. $1\frac{1}{2}$ cups to tablespoons

17. 32 fluid ounces to pints

18. 160 cups to quarts

19. 32 tablespoons to cups

20. 3 quarts to cups

Solve the following problems. After taking the test, see "Step-by-Step Solutions" for the answers (pages 306 to 308). And see "7.1 Household Measures for Length," "7.2 Household Measures for Weight," and "7.3 Household Measures for Volume" if the chapter test indicates you need additional practice.

Sections 7.1 and 7.2

*Convert the following measurements using **one** unit multiplier.*

1. 5 tablespoons to teaspoons

2. 20 inches to feet

3. $7\frac{1}{2}$ pints to cups

4. 7 tablespoons to fluid ounces

5. 18 teaspoons to tablespoons

6. 9 pints to quarts

7. 3.5 tons to pounds

8. 4.6 miles to feet

9. 14 fluid ounces to cups

10. 2,640 feet to miles

11. 3 fluid ounces to tablespoons

12. 6 quarts to gallons

13. 1.5 pounds to ounces

14. 81 feet to yards

15. 4 fluid ounces to cups

16. 12 quarts to pints

17. $3\frac{1}{2}$ feet to inches

Section 7.3

*Convert the following measurements using **two** unit multipliers.*

18. 4 pints to fluid ounces

19. 2 cups to quarts

20. 2.5 fluid ounces to teaspoons

chapter 8

The Metric System

8.0   Pretest for the Metric System

Solve the following problems. After taking the test, see "Step-by-Step Solutions" for the answers (page 309). Then, see "8.1 Multiplication and Division by Powers of 10," "8.2 Metric System Basics," "8.3 Metric Units Used in Nursing," and "8.4 Converting Units in the Metric System" for skill explanations.

Section 8.1

1. 52.467 • 100

2. 897.2 ÷ 10,000

Section 8.2

3. 1 kg = _____ g

4. 1 mm = _____ m

5. 1 g = _____ mcg

Sections 8.3 and 8.4

6. 75,000 g = _____ kg

7. 5 m = _____ cm

8. 1.4 m = _____ mm

9. 34.5 mg = _____ g

10. 5.3 mL = _____ L

In this section, we will review:
- powers of 10
- multiplying by powers of 10
- dividing by powers of 10
- moving decimal points

Powers of 10

The metric system is a base 10 system like our place value system. As you move between places in a base 10 system, you are either multiplying or dividing by a **power of 10**.

The **power of 10** is written using an exponent, which is the small number to the upper right of the 10, (10^1). The positive exponent represents the number of zeros that follow the 1, or how many times 10 has been multiplied by itself. See Table 8.1 for the powers of 10 and their meanings and values. (See also Section 5.4 Terminology for Algebra, page 127.)

Tip: To multiply and divide by powers of 10, you simply move the decimal point in the number. The answer is the same whether you choose to move the decimal point or to actually multiply or divide the numbers. Moving the decimal point is the quickest method.

Multiplying by Powers of 10

When multiplying any number by a power of 10, simply move the decimal point to the right (⇨) the indicated number of places. To determine the number of places to move the decimal point, count the number of zeros in the power of 10 and move the decimal point that many places to the right. Keep in mind that when you move a decimal point to the right (⇨) the number gets larger. These are the steps for multiplying by a power of 10:

Table 8.1	Powers of 10	
Power of 10	**Meaning**	**Value**
10 or 10^1	10	10
10^2	10 • 10	100
10^3	10 • 10 • 10	1,000
10^4	10 • 10 • 10 • 10	10,000

1. Count the number of zeros in the power of 10.
2. Draw the indicated number of small arrows to the right and place the new decimal point.
3. If needed, fill in zeros to reach the new decimal point.
4. Make certain the answer is in best mathematical form. Drop any trailing zeros.

Example 1: 36.45 • 10

STEP 1. Observe that 10 has 1 zero.

$$36.45 \bullet 10$$

STEP 2. Draw 1 arrow to the right and place the new decimal point.

$$36.4.5$$

STEP 3. Note that no additional zeros are needed.

STEP 4. Write the answer in best mathematical form.

$$364.5$$

The answer is 364.5.

Your work should look like this.

$$36.45 \bullet 10 = 36.4.5 = 364.5$$

Example 2: 574.3 • 100

STEP 1. Observe that 100 has 2 zeros.

$$574.3 \bullet 100$$

STEP 2. Draw 2 arrows to the right and place the new decimal point.

$$574.3 \,.$$

STEP 3. Fill in 1 zero to reach the new decimal point.

$$574.30.$$

STEP 4. Write the answer in best mathematical form.

$$57,430$$

The answer is 57,430.

Your work should look like this.

$$574.3 \bullet 100 = 574.30. = 57,430$$

Example 3: 276.59 • 10,000

STEP 1. Observe that 10,000 has 4 zeros.

276.59 • 10,000

STEP 2. Draw 4 arrows to the right and place the new decimal point.

276.59 .

STEP 3. Fill in 2 zeros to reach the new decimal point.

276.5900.

STEP 4. Write the answer in best mathematical form.

2,765,900

The answer is 2,765,900.

Your work should look like this.

276.59 • 10,000 = 276.5900. = 2,765,900

Dividing by Powers of 10

When dividing any number by a power of 10, simply move the decimal point to the left (⇐) the number of times indicated by the exponent. Count the number of zeros in the power of 10 and move the decimal point that number of places. Keep in mind that when you move a decimal point to the left (⇐) in a number, the number gets smaller. These are the steps for dividing by a power of 10.

1. Count the number of zeros in the power of 10. Draw the indicated number of small arrows to the left and place the new decimal point.
2. If needed, fill in zeros to reach the new decimal point.
3. Make certain the answer is in best mathematical form. For answers with only a decimal part, place a zero to the left of the decimal point.

Example 4: 31.67 ÷ 10

STEP 1. Observe that 10 has 1 zero.

31.67 ÷ 10

STEP 2. Draw 1 arrow to the left and place the new decimal point.

3.1.67

STEP 3. Note that no additional zeros are needed.

STEP 4. Write the answer in best mathematical form.

3.167

The answer is 3.167.

Your work should look like this.

31.67 ÷ 10 = 3.1.67 = 3.167

Example 5: 473.432 ÷ 10,000

STEP 1. Observe that 10,000 has 4 zeros.

473.432 ÷ 10,000

STEP 2. Draw 4 arrows to the left and place the new decimal point.

. 473.432

STEP 3. Fill in 1 zero to reach the new decimal point.

.0473.432

STEP 4. Place a zero to the left of the decimal point in answers with only a decimal part.

0.0473432

The answer is 0.0473432.

Your work should look like this.

473.432 ÷ 10,000 = .0473.432 = 0.0473432

Example 6: 0.56 ÷ 100

STEP 1. Observe that 100 has 2 zeros.

0.56 ÷ 100

STEP 2. Draw 2 arrows to the left and place the new decimal point.

. 0.56

STEP 3. Fill in 1 zero to reach the new decimal point.

.00.56

STEP 4. Place a zero to the left of the decimal point in answers with only a decimal part.

0.0056

The answer is 0.0056.

Your work should look like this on paper.

0.56 ÷ 100 = .00.56 = 0.0056

8.1 Practice Multiplying and Dividing by Powers of 10

Solve the following problems. For the answers, see "Step-by-Step Solutions" (pages 309 to 310).

1. 3.46 • 100

2. 45.61 ÷ 1,000

3. 78.4 ÷ 100

4. 0.435 • 10

5. 1.54 ÷ 10,000

6. 4.1782 • 1,000

7. 167 ÷ 10

8. 16.493 ÷ 100

9. 0.00615 • 10,000

10. 1.86 • 10

11. 20.57 • 100

12. 73.85 ÷ 1,000

13. 0.38 • 1,000

14. 157.1 ÷ 10

15. 169.9 ÷ 10,000

16. 0.719 • 10

17. 24.5 ÷ 1,000

18. 7.4 • 10,000

19. 38.2 • 100

20. 10.413 ÷ 10,000

Metric System Basics

In this section, we will review:
- metric system use
- history of the metric system
- prefixes in the metric system

Metric System Use

The **metric system** is an international standard of measurement for most of the world. The metric system is useful in naming very large and very small numbers. Although we use household measures in the United States, the metric system is the legal standard of measure in the United States.

History of the Metric System

The need for a standard worldwide unit of measure for use in areas, such as trade, scientific research, and medicine, was realized long ago. A group of scientists met in France in the 1700s to develop a unified system of measurement. Some units in the metric system were derived using the properties of the earth and water (meter and gram). Other units like the liter were derived using other metric measures. There are seven basic measures or units in the metric system. Table 8.2 explains how the group of scientists derived the metric units of measure most commonly used in nursing: the meter, gram, and liter. Note that metric abbreviations are not followed by a period.

Prefixes in the Metric System

All units of measure in the metric system use the same prefixes. Because the metric system is a base 10 system, powers of 10 represent the value of

Table 8.2	Derivation of Metric Measures	
Measure	**Symbol**	**Derivation**
meter	m	1 ten millionth (1/10,000,000) of the length of a line (meridian) beginning at the North Pole, passing through Paris, France, and ending at the equator.
gram	g	The weight of 1 cubic centimeter of water at its melting point, 4 degrees Celsius.
liter	L	The volume of a cube with each side 0.1 meter.

the different prefixes. Note that both positive and negative exponents are used to represent the prefixes in the metric system. Also notice that the metric base unit, for instance 1 gram, is located in Table 8.3 between the positive and negative exponents of 10. The power of 10 for the base unit is shown as 10^0 (10 to the zero power), which has a value of 1. By definition, any number to the zero power equals 1.

Table 8.3	**Metric System Prefixes**			
Prefix	**Symbol**	**Meaning**	**Value**	**Power of 10**
mega-	M	one million	1,000,000	10^6
hectokilo-	hk	one hundred thousand	100,000	10^5
myria-	ma	ten thousand	10,000	10^4
kilo-	k	one thousand	1,000	10^3
hecto-	h	one hundred	100	10^2
deca-	da	ten	10	10^1
BASE UNIT		one	1	10^0
deci-	d	one tenth	$\frac{1}{10}$ or 0.1	10^{-1}
centi-	c	one hundredth	$\frac{1}{100}$ or 0.01	10^{-2}
milli-	m	one thousandth	$\frac{1}{1,000}$ or 0.001	10^{-3}
decimilli-	dm	one ten thousandth	$\frac{1}{10,000}$ or 0.0001	10^{-4}
centimilli-	cm	one hundred thousandth	$\frac{1}{100,000}$ or 0.00001	10^{-5}
micro	mc	one millionth	$\frac{1}{1,000,000}$ or 0.000001	10^{-6}

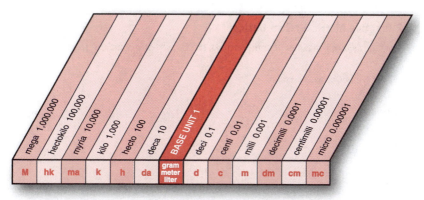

Figure 8.1: Metric system prefixes.

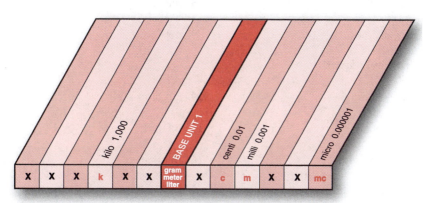

Figure 8.2: Metric prefixes used in nursing.

The metric system can be illustrated on a metric line. Understanding a metric line begins at the base unit. All places to the left of the base unit represent positive powers of 10 and indicate whole numbers ($10^1 = 10$). All places to the right of the base unit represent negative powers of 10 and indicate fractional parts of whole numbers ($10^{-1} = \frac{1}{10} = 0.1$). Figure 8.1 shows the different prefixes and values for **any** unit of measure in the metric system.

To visualize the metric prefixes most commonly used in nursing, see Figure 8.2. Gram, meter, and liter are shown as the base unit since they are the metric units most commonly used in nursing. The prefixes infrequently used are denoted with an *x*.

8.2 Practice Metric System Basics

Answer the following questions. For the answers, see "Step-by-Step Solutions" (pages 311 to 312).

Write the symbol for each prefix.

1. deca

2. milli

3. centi

4. kilo

5. micro

Write the value of each prefix.

6. centi

7. kilo

8. micro

9. milli

Which unit is larger?

10. g or mg

11. g or kg

12. mcg or g

13. m or mm

14. km or m

15. mL or L

16. m or cm

Write the value of each power of 10.

17. 10^3 = _____

18. 10^{-6} = _____

19. 10^{-3} = _____

20. 10^6 = _____

Metric Units Used in Nursing
In this section, we will review:
- three common metric units in nursing
- easy reference points for metric measures

Meter

The meter is the basic unit of length in the metric system. The length units used in nursing are the meter (m), the centimeter (cm), and the millimeter (mm).

Tip: These are reference points for meters:

- 1 meter is a little longer than a yardstick.
- 1 centimeter is the approximate diameter of a dime.
- 1 millimeter is the approximate thickness of a compact disk (CD).

Table 8.4	Meter Equivalents	
1 meter (m) = 100 centimeters (cm)	100 centimeters (cm) = 1 meter (m)
1 meter (m) = 1,000 millimeters (mm)	1,000 millimeters (mm) = 1 meter (m)
1 centimeter (cm) = 10 millimeters (mm)	10 millimeters (mm) = 1 centimeter (cm)

Figure 8.3 shows commonly used meter measurements. Keep in mind that as you move to the right of the base unit, 1 meter, the length becomes shorter.

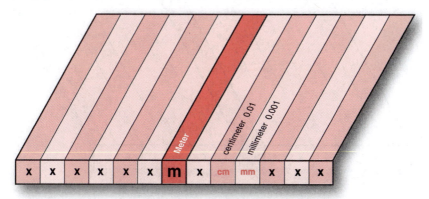

Figure 8.3: Commonly used meter measurements.

Gram

The gram is the basic unit of weight in the metric system. The weight units used in nursing are the kilogram (kg), gram (g), milligram (mg), and microgram (mcg).

Tip: These are reference points for grams:

- 1 kilogram is the weight of slightly more than a quart of water.
- 1 gram is the weight of a paper clip.
- 1 milligram is the weight of a pinch of salt.
- 1 microgram is the weight of something too small to see.

Table 8.5	Gram Equivalents	
1 kilogram (kg) = 1,000 grams (g)	1,000 grams (g) = 1 kilogram (kg)
1 gram (g) = 1,000 milligrams (mg)	1,000 milligrams (mg) = 1 gram (g)
1 gram (g) = 1,000,000 micrograms (mcg)	1,000,000 micrograms (mcg) = 1 gram (g)
1 milligram (mg) = 1,000 micrograms	1,000 micrograms (mcg) = 1 milligram (mg)

Figure 8.4 shows commonly used gram measurements. Keep in mind that as you move to the left of the base unit, 1 gram, the weight increases. As you move to the right of the unit, the weight decreases.

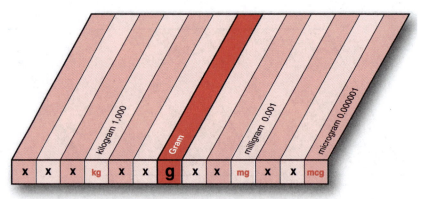

Figure 8.4: Commonly used gram measurements.

Liter

The liter is the basic unit of volume in the metric system. The units of volume used in nursing are the liter (L) and the milliliter (mL).

Tip: These are reference points for liters:

- 1 liter is a little more than 1 quart.
- 1 milliliter is approximately 1 drip from a faucet.

Table 8.6	Liter Equivalents	
1 liter (L) = 1,000 milliliters (mL)		1,000 milliliters (mL) = 1 liter (L)
1 milliliter (mL) = 1 cubic centimeter (cm³)*		1 cubic centimeter (cm³) = 1 milliliter (mL)

* The abbreviation cc for cubic centimeter recently has been prohibited in the health-care industry because cc is easily mistaken for two zeros.

Figure 8.5 shows commonly used liter measurements. Keep in mind that as you move to the right of the base unit, 1 liter, the volume decreases.

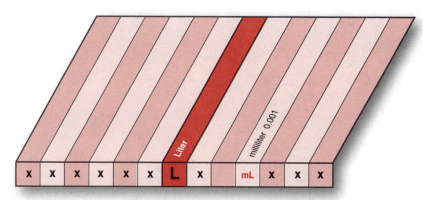

Figure 8.5: Commonly used liter measurements.

8.3 Practice Metric Units Used in Nursing

Solve the following problems. For the answers, see "Step-by-Step Solutions" (pages 312 to 313).
State the reference point for the following metric units.

1. 1 meter

2. 1 centimeter

3. 1 gram

4. 1 milligram

5. 1 millimeter

6. 1 kilogram

7. 1 milliliter

Convert these measurements.

8. 1 g = _____ mg

9. 1,000 g = _____ kg

10. 0.000001 g = _____ mcg

11. 1 mg = _____ mcg

12. 1 km = _____ m

13. 1,000,000 mcg = _____ g

14. 1 m = _____ cm

15. 1,000 mL = _____ L

16. 1 mg = _____ g

17. 1 m = _____ km

18. 1 mm = _____ cm

19. 1,000 mm = _____ m

20. 1 cm = _____ m

Converting Units in the Metric System
In this section, we will review:
- converting metric units by visualizing the metric line
- converting metric units by considering the size of the unit

Converting Metric Units by Visualizing the Metric Line

Making conversions in the metric system requires multiplying or dividing by powers of 10. The conversions are made by moving the decimal point to the right or left. Metric conversions can be performed by visualizing the metric line. Memorizing prefix values and visualizing unit placement on a metric line is essential. The location on the metric line of the two units in a conversion problem determines whether you move the decimal point to the right or to the left.

See Figure 8.6 (Metric prefixes used in nursing). Recall, that the x denotes prefixes infrequently used.

Here are the steps to visually perform a metric conversion.

1. Visualize the measure you are given and the desired measure on the metric line or draw a simple sketch of the line.
2. Start at the measure you are given.
3. If the desired unit of measure is to the left of the given unit, move the decimal point to the left that number of places.
4. If the desired unit of measure is to the right of the given unit, move the decimal point to the right that number of places.

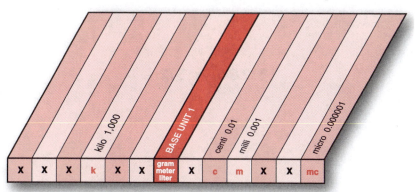

Figure 8.6: Metric prefixes commonly used in nursing.

Converting Metric Units by Considering the Size of the Unit

Rule 1: If converting **larger** units to **smaller** units, **multiply** to move the decimal point to the right ($\Rightarrow$). Why multiply? Because more small units are needed to equal a large one. Count the number of decimal places to reach the desired unit. Place the decimal point, and fill in zeros, if needed.

Rule 2: If converting **smaller** units to **larger** units, **divide**, to move the decimal point to the left ($\Leftarrow$). Why divide? Because less of a larger unit is needed to equal a smaller unit. Count the number of decimal places to reach the desired unit. Place the decimal point, and fill in zeros, if needed. Remember to remove trailing zeros.

The examples in this section use a combination of the visual and size methods combined. You will need to determine which method works best for you.

Example 1: 3,200 mL = __ L

STEP 1. Visualize mL and L on the metric line. Milliliters are smaller than liters, so you need to divide (move left).

$\longleftarrow$
L mL

STEP 2. Recall the conversion 1,000 mL = 1 L. Move the decimal point to the left 3 places since 1,000 = 10^3.

3.200.

STEP 3. Remove the trailing zeros.

3.2

The answer is 3.2 L.

Your work should look like this.

3.200. = 3.2 L

Example 2: 3.94 g = ___ mg

STEP 1. Visualize grams and mg on the metric line. Grams are larger than milligrams, so you need to multiply (move right).

→

g mg

STEP 2. Recall the conversion 1 gram = 1,000 mg. Move the decimal point 3 places to the right since 1,000 = 10^3.

3.94 .

STEP 3. Fill in 1 zero to reach the new decimal point.

3,940

The answer is 3,940 mg.

Your work should look like this on paper.

3.940. = 3,940 mg

Example 3: 3.1 cm = ___ mm

STEP 1. Visualize centimeters and millimeters on the metric line. Centimeters are larger than millimeters, so you need to multiply (move right).

→

cm mm

STEP 2. Recall the conversion 1 cm = 10 mm. Move the decimal point 1 place to the right since 10 = 10^1.

3.1.

STEP 3. Notice that the answer is in best form.

31

The answer is 31 mm.

Your work should look like this on paper.

3.1. = 31 mm

Example 4:   4,500 mm = _____ m

STEP 1. Visualize mm and m on the metric line. Millimeters are smaller than meters, so you need to divide (move left).

←

m mm

STEP 2. Recall the conversion 1,000 mm = 1 m. Move the decimal point to the left 3 places since $1,000 = 10^3$.

4.500.

STEP 3. Remove the trailing zeros.

4.5

The answer is 4.5 m.

Your answer should look like this.

4.500. = 4.5 m

8.4 Practice Converting Units in the Metric System

Solve the following problems. For the answers, see "Step-by-Step Solutions" (pages 313 to 316).

See Figure 8.6.

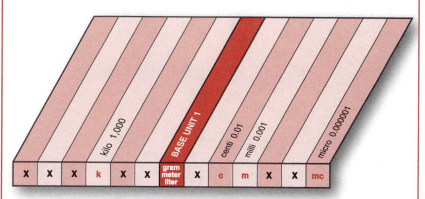

Figure 8.6: Metric prefixes commonly used in nursing.

Use the metric line above to help visualize and perform the conversions.

1. 12 m = _____ cm

2. 34.6 g = _____ mg

3. 48 mm = _____ m

4. 75 mcg = _____ mg

5. 735 mg = _____ g

6. 2 mL = _____ L

7. 0.3 m = _____ mm

8. 73 kg = _____ mg

9. 3.4 L = _____ mL

10. 6.4 cm = _____ m

11. 7,480 g = _____ kg

12. 536 cm³ = _____ mL

13. 2 mcg = _____ mg

14. 528 cm = _____ m

15. 50 L = _____ mL

16. 0.54 g = _____ mg

17. 12 mg = _____ mcg

18. 2.27 mL = _____ L

19. 25 mm = _____ cm

20. 896 g = _____ mg

Solve the following problems. After taking the test, see "Step-by-Step Solutions" for the answers (pages 316 to 318). And see "8.1 Multiplication and Division by Powers of 10," "8.2 Metric System Basics," "8.3 Metric Units Used in Nursing," and "8.4 Converting Units in the Metric System" if the chapter test indicates you need additional practice.

Section 8.1

1. $27.45 \bullet 1{,}000$

2. $0.23 \div 10$

3. $15.642 \bullet 100$

4. $9.1 \div 10{,}000$

Section 8.2

5. kilo has a value of _____

6. centi has a value of _____

7. milli has a value of _____

8. micro has a value of _____

Sections 8.3 and 8.4

9. $1 \ cm^3 =$ _____ mL

10. 275 mcg = _____ mg

11. 135 mg = _____ g

12. 3.1 cm = _____ mm

13. 2 mg = _____ mcg

14. 2.5 kg = _____ g

15. 569 mL = _____ L

16. 0.8 mcg = _____ mg

17. 6.37 mL = _____ L

18. 5,600 g = _____ kg

19. 3.2 L = _____ mL

20. 0.3 g = _____ mcg

Practice Tests
for Measures

Fill in the blank to complete the basic unit conversions for the household and metric system. For speed and accuracy, memorize these conversions.

For test answers, see "Step-by-Step Solutions," page 319. To the left of each solution, you will notice two numbers. These numbers indicate the chapter and section—for example, (7.1) means Chapter 7, Section 1—where you can find a detailed explanation for solving similar problems. If your answer is incorrect and you need more practice, you may wish to review the indicated material.

1. 1 m = _____ cm

2. 1 ton = _____ lbs.

3. 1 cup = _____ fl. oz.

4. 1 kg = _____ g

5. 12 in. = _____ ft.

6. 1 T = _____ tsp.

7. 1,000 mm = _____ m

8. 1 mi. = _____ ft.

9. 10 mm = _____ cm

10. 2 pts. = _____ qt.

11. 2 T = _____ fl. oz.

12. 0.001 g = _____ mg

13. 1 yd. = _____ ft.

14. 1 lb. = _____ oz.

15. 1,000,000 mcg = _____ g

16. 1 gal. = _____ qt.

17. 27 cm^3 = _____ mL

18. 1 L = _____ mL

19. 1 pt. = _____ cups

20. 1 mcg = _____ g

Practice Test 2
Performing Household and Metric Conversions

Use 1 or 2 unit multipliers to complete the following household measure conversions.

For test answers, see "Step-by-Step Solutions," pages 320 to 326. To the left of each solution, you will notice two numbers. These numbers indicate the chapter and section—for example, (7.1) means Chapter 7, Section 1—where you can find a detailed explanation for solving similar problems. If your answer is incorrect and you need more practice, you may wish to review the indicated material.

1. 84 in. = _____ ft.

2. 31 pt. = _____ cups

3. 2 gal. = _____ pt.

4. 41 yd. = _____ ft.

5. 12 T. = _____ cups

6. 3 cups = _____ fl. oz.

7. 10,560 ft. = _____ mi.

8. 8 fl. oz. = _____ T.

9. $2\frac{1}{2}$ qt. _____ cups

10. 6 gal. = _____ qt.

11. 2 qt. = _____ pt.

12. 17 ft. = _____ in.

13. 14 fl. oz. = _____ pt.

14. 9 tsp. = _____ T.

15. 2 pt. = _____ fl. oz.

16. 13 tons = _____ lb.

17. 10 T. =_____ fl. oz.

18. 12 ft. = _____ yd.

19. 8 fl. oz. = _____ pt.

20. 4 lb. = _____ oz.

21. 18 pt. = _____ qt.

22. 2 cups = _____ fl. oz.

23. 144 oz. = _____ lb.

24. 32 fl. oz. = _____ cups

25. 31,680 ft. = _____ mi.

26. 54 cups = _____ pt.

27. $\frac{7}{8}$ pt. = _____ fl. oz.

28. 180 in. = _____ ft.

29. 28 qt. = _____ gal.

30. 6 T. = _____ tsp.

31. 2 fl. oz. = _____ T.

32. 4 qt. = _____ cups

33. 34,000 lb. = _____ tons

Perform the following metric conversions.

34. 46.8 m = _____ cm

35. 3.162 kg = _____ g

36. 27 mm = _____ m

37. 426 mcg = _____ mg

38. 3.82 L = _____ mL

39. 98.6 cm = _____ mm

40. 75 mL = _____ cm^3

41. 0.568 g = _____ mg

42. 0.014 g = _____ mcg

43. 5,300 mL = _____ L

44. 5,296 mm = _____ cm

45. 13 mg = _____ g

46. 294 g = _____ kg

47. 42.8 cm = _____ m

48. 0.328 m = _____ mm

49. 10 mcg = _____ g

50. 5 cm^3 = _____ mL

51. 0.25 mg = _____ mcg

52. 0.0975 mcg = _____ mg

53. 0.825 m = _____ cm

54. 45 cm^3 = _____ mL

55. 2 g = _____ mcg

56. 27 mg = _____ g

57. 37 cm = _____ mm

58. 493 L = _____ mL

59. 2.92 kg = _____ g

60. 508 mm = _____ m

1.0　　　　Pretest for Whole Numbers

Section 1.1

1.　$\overset{1\ 1}{5{,}057}$
　$+\ 8{,}876$
　$\overline{13{,}933}$

2.　$\overset{11\ 11}{12{,}672}$
　$+\ 9{,}458$
　$\overline{22{,}130}$

Section 1.2

3.　$\overset{\overset{\overset{3\ 15}{5\ 12}}{2\ 12}}{\cancel{4{,}63}2}$
　$-\ 743$
　$\overline{3{,}8\ 89}$

4.　$\overset{\overset{\overset{6\ 10}{0\ 10}}{3\ 13}}{\cancel{71}{,}043}$
　$-\ 68{,}736$
　$\overline{2{,}307}$

Section 1.3

5.　$\overset{7\ 7}{578}$
　$\times\ 9$
　$\overline{5{,}202}$

6.　$\overset{\overset{1\ 3}{2\ 4}}{625}$
　$\times\ 79$
　$\overline{\overset{1}{5}625}$
　4375
　$\overline{49{,}375}$

7.　$\overset{\overset{3\ 3}{3\ 4}}{645}$
　$\times\ 708$
　$\overline{5160}$
　45150
　$\overline{456{,}660}$

Section 1.4

8.　$\overset{\overset{2}{2}}{17\overline{)759}}\ 44\,\text{r}.11$
　$\underline{-68}$
　79
　$\underline{-68}$
　11

9.　$\overset{\overset{4}{\overset{1}{2}}}{15\overline{)8{,}080}}\ 538\,\text{r}.10$
　$\underline{-75}$
　58
　$\underline{-45}$
　130
　$\underline{-120}$
　10

10.　$\overset{\overset{1\ 2}{1\ 2}}{236\overline{)10{,}400}}\ 44\,\text{r}.16$
　$\underline{-944}$
　960
　$\underline{-944}$
　16

1.1 Practice Adding Whole Numbers

1.　408
　$+\ 241$
　$\overline{649}$

2.　523
　$+\ 271$
　$\overline{794}$

3.　405
　$+\ 561$
　$\overline{966}$

4.　216
　$+\ 423$
　$\overline{639}$

5.   640
   + 118
   758

6.   ^{1 11} 7,244
   + 2,786
   10,030

7.   ^{1 11} 8,563
   + 4,567
   13,130

8.   ^{1 1} 5,042
   + 1,966
   7,008

9.   ^{1 11} 5,787
   + 2,344
   8,131

10.   ^{1 11} 3,329
   + 4,783
   8,112

11.   ^{1 11} 4,815
   + 6,396
   11,211

12.   ^{1 11} 7,586
   + 1,645
   9,231

13.   ¹ 4,116
   + 3,168
   7,284

14.   7,121
   + 2,850
   9,971

15.   ^{1 1} 2,351
   + 7,499
   9,850

16.   ^{1 2 1} 4,386
     3,798
   + 1,745
   9,929

17.   ^{1 1} 7,038
     1,056
   + 2,784
   10,878

18.   ^{2 1 1} 6,748
     5,902
   + 4,352
   17,002

19.   ^{2 2 2} 8,764
     9,989
   + 6,478
   25,231

20.   ^{1 1 1} 2,697
     7,507
   + 4,572
   14,776

1.2 Practice Subtracting Whole Numbers

1.   7,642
  − 4,210
  3,432

2.   8,235
  − 3,123
  5,112

3.   ^{6 14} 1⁷4
  − 48
  126

4.   ^{3 17} 3⁴7
  − 129
  218

5.   ^{8 12} 6⁹2
  − 217
  475

6.   ^{7 13} ^{3 13} 7,8⁴3
  − 6,274
  1,569

7.   ^{3 13} ^{6 16} 4,3⁷6
  − 2,808
  1,568

8.   ^{2 12} 3,275
  − 1,744
  1,531

9.   ^{2 14} ^{4 16} 3,4⁵6
  − 2,738
  718

10.   ^{9 10} ^{2 10} ^{0 10} 3,0⁴0
  − 2,563
  447

11.   ^{6 11} ^{2 13} 7,133
  − 2,924
  4,209

12.   ^{4 12} ^{9 11} ^{2 10} 5,301
  − 3,466
  1,835

13.   ^{9 10} ^{1 10} 2,007
  − 347
  1,660

14.   ^{5 12} 6,231
  − 430
  5,801

15.   ^{9 10} ^{4 10} 5,005
  − 4,835
  170

16.   ^{8 10} ^{0 10} ^{0 12} 9,112
  − 2,569
  6,543

17.
$$\begin{array}{r} \scriptstyle 9\ 12 \\ \scriptstyle 9\ \cancel{10} \\ \scriptstyle 5\ \cancel{10} \\ 6{,}0\ 0\ 2 \\ -\ 3{,}5\ 74 \\ \hline 2{,}4\ 2\ 8 \end{array}$$

18.
$$\begin{array}{r} \scriptstyle 9\ 13 \\ \scriptstyle 2\ \cancel{10} \\ 8{,}3\ 03 \\ -\ 1{,}2\ 27 \\ \hline 7{,}0\ 76 \end{array}$$

19.
$$\begin{array}{r} \scriptstyle 9\ 14 \\ \scriptstyle 8\ \cancel{10} \\ 9{,}0\ 41 \\ -\ 2{,}961 \\ \hline 6{,}0\ 80 \end{array}$$

20.
$$\begin{array}{r} \scriptstyle 9\ 10 \\ \scriptstyle 9\ \cancel{10} \\ \scriptstyle 3\ \cancel{10} \\ 4{,}0\ 0\ 0 \\ -\ 2{,}5\ 64 \\ \hline 1{,}4\ 36 \end{array}$$

1.3 Practice Multiplying Whole Numbers

1.
$$\begin{array}{r} \scriptstyle 1 \\ \scriptstyle 4 \\ 36 \\ \times\ 27 \\ \hline 252 \\ 72 \\ \hline 972 \end{array}$$

2.
$$\begin{array}{r} \scriptstyle 3 \\ \scriptstyle 1 \\ 39 \\ \times\ 42 \\ \hline {}_1 78 \\ 156 \\ \hline 1{,}638 \end{array}$$

3.
$$\begin{array}{r} \scriptstyle 2\ 2 \\ \scriptstyle 1\ 1 \\ 255 \\ \times\ 43 \\ \hline 765 \\ 1020 \\ \hline 10{,}965 \end{array}$$

4.
$$\begin{array}{r} \scriptstyle 5\ 3 \\ \scriptstyle 7\ 4 \\ 895 \\ \times\ 68 \\ \hline {}_1 7160 \\ 5370 \\ \hline 60{,}860 \end{array}$$

5.
$$\begin{array}{r} \scriptstyle 1\ 2 \\ \scriptstyle 2\ 2 \\ 623 \\ \times\ 79 \\ \hline {}_1 5607 \\ 4361 \\ \hline 49{,}217 \end{array}$$

6.
$$\begin{array}{r} \scriptstyle 1\ 41 \\ \scriptstyle 2 \\ 9{,}173 \\ \times\ 63 \\ \hline 27519 \\ 55038 \\ \hline 577{,}899 \end{array}$$

7.
$$\begin{array}{r} \scriptstyle 2\ 26 \\ \scriptstyle 2 \\ 4{,}329 \\ \times\ 73 \\ \hline {}^{1\ 1} 12\,987 \\ 303\,03 \\ \hline 316{,}017 \end{array}$$

8.
$$\begin{array}{r} \scriptstyle 1 \\ \scriptstyle 1\ 15 \\ 4{,}218 \\ \times\ 27 \\ \hline {}_1 29\,526 \\ 84\,36 \\ \hline 113{,}886 \end{array}$$

9.
$$\begin{array}{r} \scriptstyle 1\ \ 1 \\ \scriptstyle 2\ \ 3 \\ \scriptstyle 2\ \ 2 \\ 7{,}516 \\ \times\ 254 \\ \hline {}_1 30\,064 \\ 375\,80 \\ 1\,503\,2 \\ \hline 1{,}909{,}064 \end{array}$$

10.
$$\begin{array}{r} \scriptstyle 5\ 2 \\ \scriptstyle 2\ 1 \\ \scriptstyle 6\ 3 \\ 784 \\ \times\ 638 \\ \hline {}_1 6272 \\ {}_1 2352 \\ 4704 \\ \hline 500{,}192 \end{array}$$

11.
$$\begin{array}{r} 71 \\ \times\ 80 \\ \hline 5{,}680 \end{array}$$

12.
$$\begin{array}{r} 62 \\ \times\ 40 \\ \hline 2{,}480 \end{array}$$

13.
$$\begin{array}{r} 31 \\ \times\ 90 \\ \hline 2{,}790 \end{array}$$

14.
$$\begin{array}{r} \scriptstyle 1 \\ 471 \\ \times\ 20 \\ \hline 9{,}420 \end{array}$$

15.
$$\begin{array}{r} \scriptstyle 2 \\ 891 \\ \times\ 30 \\ \hline 26{,}730 \end{array}$$

16.
$$\begin{array}{r} 710 \\ \times\ 806 \\ \hline {}_1 4260 \\ 56800 \\ \hline 572{,}260 \end{array}$$

17.
$$\begin{array}{r} 123 \\ \times\ 302 \\ \hline {}_1 246 \\ 3690 \\ \hline 37{,}146 \end{array}$$

18.
$$\begin{array}{r} 1{,}002 \\ \times\ 123 \\ \hline 3006 \\ 2004 \\ 1002 \\ \hline 123{,}246 \end{array}$$

19.
$$\begin{array}{r} 801 \\ \times\ 497 \\ \hline {}_1 5607 \\ 7209 \\ 3204 \\ \hline 398{,}097 \end{array}$$

20.
$$\begin{array}{r} 4{,}020 \\ \times\ 202 \\ \hline {}_1 8040 \\ 80400 \\ \hline 812{,}040 \end{array}$$

1.4 Practice Dividing Whole Numbers

1.
$$\begin{array}{r} 6 \\ 8\overline{)48} \\ \underline{-48} \\ 0 \end{array}$$

2.
$$\begin{array}{r} 7 \\ 7\overline{)49} \\ \underline{-49} \\ 0 \end{array}$$

3.
$$\begin{array}{r} 9\,r.4 \\ 9\overline{)85} \\ \underline{-81} \\ 4 \end{array}$$

4.
$$\begin{array}{r} 4\,r.2 \\ 5\overline{)22} \\ \underline{-20} \\ 2 \end{array}$$

5.
$$\begin{array}{r} {}^{3}_{1}\quad 24\,r.23 \\ 28\overline{)695} \\ \underline{-56} \\ 135 \\ \underline{-112} \\ 23 \end{array}$$

6.
$$\begin{array}{r} {}_{4}\quad 8 \\ 16\overline{)128} \\ \underline{-128} \\ 0 \end{array}$$

7.
$$\begin{array}{r} 15\,r.5 \\ 20\overline{)305} \\ \underline{-20} \\ 105 \\ \underline{-100} \\ 5 \end{array}$$

8.
$$\begin{array}{r} {}_{2}\quad 3\,r.3 \\ 68\overline{)207} \\ \underline{-204} \\ 3 \end{array}$$

9.
$$\begin{array}{r} {}_{1}\quad 20 \\ 17\overline{)340} \\ \underline{-34} \\ 00 \\ \underline{-0} \\ 0 \end{array}$$

10.
$$\begin{array}{r} {}_{1}\quad 20\,r.13 \\ 49\overline{)993} \\ \underline{-98} \\ 13 \\ \underline{-0} \\ 13 \end{array}$$

11.
$$\begin{array}{r} {}_{3}\quad 400\,r.3 \\ 19\overline{)7,603} \\ \underline{-76} \\ 00 \\ \underline{-0} \\ 03 \\ \underline{-0} \\ 3 \end{array}$$

12.
$$\begin{array}{r} 301\,r.4 \\ 13\overline{)3,917} \\ \underline{-39} \\ 01 \\ \underline{-0} \\ 17 \\ \underline{-13} \\ 4 \end{array}$$

13.
$$\begin{array}{r} 933\,r.26 \\ 51\overline{)47,609} \\ \underline{-459} \\ 170 \\ \underline{-153} \\ 179 \\ \underline{-153} \\ 26 \end{array}$$

14.
$$\begin{array}{r} {}^{2}_{1}\quad 205 \\ 95\overline{)19,475} \\ \underline{-190} \\ 47 \\ \underline{-0} \\ 475 \\ \underline{-475} \\ 0 \end{array}$$

15.
$$\begin{array}{r} {}^{1}_{1}\quad 1,022\,r.44 \\ 89\overline{)91,002} \\ \underline{-89} \\ 20 \\ \underline{-0} \\ 200 \\ \underline{-178} \\ 222 \\ \underline{-178} \\ 44 \end{array}$$

16.
$$\begin{array}{r} {}_{2}\quad 7\,r.358 \\ 630\overline{)4,768} \\ \underline{-4410} \\ 358 \end{array}$$

17.
$$\begin{array}{r} {}_{2}\quad 4\,r.192 \\ 716\overline{)3,056} \\ \underline{-2864} \\ 192 \end{array}$$

18.
$$\begin{array}{r} {}^{1}_{1}\quad 196\,r.370 \\ 502\overline{)98,762} \\ \underline{-502} \\ 4856 \\ \underline{-4518} \\ 3382 \\ \underline{-3012} \\ 370 \end{array}$$

19.
$$\begin{array}{r} {}^{3}_{2}\quad 68\,r.224 \\ 741\overline{)50,612} \\ \underline{-4446} \\ 6152 \\ \underline{-5928} \\ 224 \end{array}$$

20.
$$\begin{array}{r} {}^{77}_{44}\quad 1,058\,r.514 \\ 789\overline{)835,276} \\ \underline{-789} \\ 462 \\ \underline{-0} \\ 4627 \\ \underline{-3945} \\ 6826 \\ \underline{-6312} \\ 514 \end{array}$$

1.5 Chapter Test for Whole Numbers

Section 1.1

1.
$$\begin{array}{r} {\scriptstyle 1\,1} \\ 7{,}203 \\ +\ 9{,}097 \\ \hline 16{,}300 \end{array}$$

2.
$$\begin{array}{r} {\scriptstyle 1\ 11} \\ 12{,}594 \\ +\ 6{,}789 \\ \hline 19{,}383 \end{array}$$

3.
$$\begin{array}{r} {\scriptstyle 1\ 1} \\ 70{,}698 \\ +\ 5{,}921 \\ \hline 76{,}619 \end{array}$$

4.
$$\begin{array}{r} {\scriptstyle 1} \\ 5{,}742 \\ +\ 8{,}706 \\ \hline 14{,}448 \end{array}$$

5.
$$\begin{array}{r} {\scriptstyle 1\,1} \\ 39{,}424 \\ +\ 65{,}875 \\ \hline 105{,}299 \end{array}$$

Section 1.2

6.
$$\begin{array}{r} {\scriptstyle 4\ \ 16} \\ {\scriptstyle 6\ 10} \\ 5{,}7\,0\,4 \\ -\ \ 8\,9\,2 \\ \hline 4{,}8\,1\,2 \end{array}$$

7.
$$\begin{array}{r} {\scriptstyle 5\ \ 11} \\ {\scriptstyle 1\ 12} \\ {\scriptstyle 2\ 11} \\ 6{,}2\,3\,1 \\ -\ 1{,}5\,7\,6 \\ \hline 4{,}6\,5\,5 \end{array}$$

8.
$$\begin{array}{r} {\scriptstyle 0\,12} \\ {\scriptstyle 2\ \ 13} \\ {\scriptstyle 3\ 15} \\ 13{,}4\,5\,2 \\ -\ 9{,}5\,7\,1 \\ \hline 3{,}8\,8\,1 \end{array}$$

9.
$$\begin{array}{r} {\scriptstyle 9\ 14} \\ {\scriptstyle 9\ 10} \\ {\scriptstyle 4\ 10} \\ 7\,5{,}0\,0\,4 \\ -\,7\,4{,}9\,8\,9 \\ \hline 1\ 5 \end{array}$$

10.
$$\begin{array}{r} {\scriptstyle 9\ 10} \\ {\scriptstyle 9\ 10} \\ {\scriptstyle 9\ 10} \\ {\scriptstyle 8\ 10} \\ 9\,0{,}0\,0\,0 \\ -\,7\,1{,}2\,3\,4 \\ \hline 1\,8{,}7\,6\,6 \end{array}$$

Section 1.3

11.
$$\begin{array}{r} {\scriptstyle 2\,2} \\ 734 \\ \times\ \ \ 7 \\ \hline 5{,}138 \end{array}$$

12.
$$\begin{array}{r} {\scriptstyle 1\,1} \\ {\scriptstyle 3\,2} \\ 576 \\ \times\ 24 \\ \hline 2\,304 \\ 11\,52\ \ \\ \hline 13{,}824 \end{array}$$

13.
$$\begin{array}{r} 702 \\ \times\ 30 \\ \hline 21{,}060 \end{array}$$

14.
$$\begin{array}{r} {\scriptstyle 2\ \ 4} \\ {\scriptstyle 3\ \ 6} \\ 9{,}407 \\ \times\ 609 \\ \hline {\scriptstyle 1}84663 \\ 564420\ \ \\ \hline 5{,}728{,}863 \end{array}$$

15.
$$\begin{array}{r} {\scriptstyle 1\ \ 31} \\ 12{,}072 \\ \times\ 1{,}005 \\ \hline {\scriptstyle 1}60360 \\ 1207200\ \ \ \\ \hline 12{,}132{,}360 \end{array}$$

Section 1.4

16.
$$
\begin{array}{r}
\overset{3}{}\quad 6\ \text{r.19} \\
26\overline{)175} \\
\underline{-156} \\
19
\end{array}
$$

17.
$$
\begin{array}{r}
\overset{7}{}\quad 8\ \text{r.51} \\
79\overline{)683} \\
\underline{-632} \\
51
\end{array}
$$

18.
$$
\begin{array}{r}
\overset{3\,3}{\underset{2\,2}{}}\quad 46\ \text{r.700} \\
756\overline{)35{,}476} \\
\underline{-3024} \\
5236 \\
\underline{-4536} \\
700
\end{array}
$$

19.
$$
\begin{array}{r}
\overset{3\,1}{\underset{1}{}}\quad 39\ \text{r.371} \\
642\overline{)25{,}409} \\
\underline{-1926} \\
6149 \\
\underline{-5778} \\
371
\end{array}
$$

20.
$$
\begin{array}{r}
\overset{3}{\underset{3}{7}}\quad 494\ \text{r.262} \\
708\overline{)350{,}014} \\
\underline{-2832} \\
6681 \\
\underline{-6372} \\
3094 \\
\underline{-2832} \\
262
\end{array}
$$

2.0 Pretest for Fractions

Section 2.1

1. $\dfrac{50}{4}$

$\begin{array}{r} 12\frac{2}{4} = 12\frac{1}{2} \\ 4\overline{)50} \\ \underline{-4} \\ 10 \\ \underline{-8} \\ 2 \end{array}$

2. $6\dfrac{7}{8} = \dfrac{\overset{48}{(6 \times 8)} + 7}{8} = \dfrac{55}{8}$

Section 2.2

3. $\dfrac{\overset{1}{\cancel{4}}}{\underset{1}{\cancel{7}}} \times \dfrac{\overset{4}{\cancel{28}}}{\underset{9}{\cancel{36}}} = \dfrac{4}{9}$

4. $5\dfrac{7}{9} \times 3\dfrac{4}{13} = \dfrac{\overset{4}{\cancel{52}}}{9} \times \dfrac{43}{\underset{1}{\cancel{13}}} = \dfrac{172}{9}$

$\begin{array}{r} 19\frac{1}{9} \\ 9\overline{)172} \\ \underline{-9} \\ 82 \\ \underline{-81} \\ 1 \end{array}$

Section 2.3

5. $\dfrac{9}{14} \div \dfrac{3}{21} = \dfrac{\overset{3}{\cancel{9}}}{\underset{2}{\cancel{14}}} \times \dfrac{\overset{3}{\cancel{21}}}{\underset{1}{\cancel{3}}} = \dfrac{9}{2}$

$\begin{array}{r} 4\frac{1}{2} \\ 2\overline{)9} \\ \underline{-8} \\ 1 \end{array}$

6. $5\dfrac{3}{5} \div 2\dfrac{6}{25} = \dfrac{28}{5} \div \dfrac{56}{25} = \dfrac{\overset{1}{\underset{1}{\cancel{28}}}}{\underset{1}{\cancel{5}}} \times \dfrac{\overset{5}{\cancel{25}}}{\underset{2}{\cancel{56}}} = \dfrac{5}{2} = 2\dfrac{1}{2}$

Sections 2.4 and 2.5

7.
$\begin{array}{r} 5\frac{3}{5} \bullet \frac{3}{3} = 5\frac{9}{15} \\ + 7\frac{4}{15} = + 7\frac{4}{15} \\ \hline 12\frac{13}{15} \end{array}$

$LCD = 5 \bullet 1 \bullet 3 = 15$

$\begin{array}{c} 5\overline{)5 \quad 15} \\ 1 \quad 3 \end{array}$

8. $\dfrac{1}{5} + \dfrac{3}{8} + \dfrac{7}{10}$

LCD $= 2 \bullet 5 \bullet 1 \bullet 4 \bullet 1 = 40$

$$\begin{array}{c|ccc} 2 & 5 & 8 & 10 \\ 5 & 5 & 4 & 5 \\ & 1 & 4 & 1 \end{array}$$

$\dfrac{1}{5} \bullet \dfrac{8}{8} = \dfrac{8}{40}$

$\dfrac{3}{8} \bullet \dfrac{5}{5} = \dfrac{15}{40}$

$+ \dfrac{7}{10} \bullet \dfrac{4}{4} = \dfrac{28}{40}$

$\dfrac{51}{40} = 1\dfrac{11}{40}$

$$40\overline{)51}^{\,1\frac{11}{40}}$$
$$\dfrac{-40}{11}$$

Sections 2.4 and 2.6

9. $\dfrac{7}{22} - \dfrac{3}{11}$ LCD $= 11 \bullet 2 \bullet 1 = 22$

$$\begin{array}{c|cc} 11 & 22 & 11 \\ & 2 & 1 \end{array}$$

$\dfrac{7}{22} \quad = \quad \dfrac{7}{22}$

$- \dfrac{3}{11} \bullet \dfrac{2}{2} = - \dfrac{6}{22}$

$\dfrac{1}{22}$

10.

$14\dfrac{5}{8} \bullet \dfrac{7}{7} = \quad 1\cancel{4}\dfrac{35}{56} = 13\dfrac{91}{56}$ $\left(3\dfrac{56}{56}\right)$

$- 5\dfrac{9}{14} \bullet \dfrac{4}{4} = \quad - 5\dfrac{36}{56} = - 5\dfrac{36}{56}$

$8\dfrac{55}{56}$

LCD $= 2 \bullet 4 \bullet 7 = 56$

$$\begin{array}{c|cc} 2 & 8 & 14 \\ & 4 & 7 \end{array}$$

2.1 Practice Fraction Terminology

1. $28 = \dfrac{28}{1}$

2. $72 = \dfrac{72}{1}$

3. $\dfrac{16}{3} = 5\dfrac{1}{3}$

$$3\overline{)16}^{\,5\frac{1}{3}}$$
$$\dfrac{-15}{1}$$

4. $\dfrac{23}{5} = 4\dfrac{3}{5}$

$$5\overline{)23}^{\,4\frac{3}{5}}$$
$$\dfrac{-20}{3}$$

5. $\dfrac{35}{4} = 8\dfrac{3}{4}$

$$4\overline{)35}^{\,8\frac{3}{4}}$$
$$\dfrac{-32}{3}$$

6. $\dfrac{61}{8} = 7\dfrac{5}{8}$

$$8\overline{)61}^{\,7\frac{5}{8}}$$
$$\dfrac{-56}{5}$$

7. $\dfrac{49}{4} = 12\dfrac{1}{4}$ $4\overline{)49}$ → $12\dfrac{1}{4}$
$\dfrac{-4}{09}$
$\dfrac{-8}{1}$

8. $10\dfrac{1}{3} = \dfrac{(10 \overset{30}{\times} 3)+1}{3} = \dfrac{31}{3}$

9. $7\dfrac{5}{8} = \dfrac{(7 \overset{56}{\times} 8)+5}{8} = \dfrac{61}{8}$

10. $9\dfrac{1}{2} = \dfrac{(9 \overset{18}{\times} 2)+1}{2} = \dfrac{19}{2}$

11. $2\dfrac{9}{10} = \dfrac{(2 \overset{20}{\times} 10)+9}{10} = \dfrac{29}{10}$

12. $4\dfrac{5}{12} = \dfrac{(4 \overset{48}{\times} 12)+5}{12} = \dfrac{53}{12}$

13. $\dfrac{4}{12} = \dfrac{\overset{1}{\cancel{2}} \times 2}{\underset{1}{\cancel{2}} \times 6} = \dfrac{2}{6} = \dfrac{1 \times \overset{1}{\cancel{2}}}{\underset{1}{\cancel{2}} \times 3} = \dfrac{1}{3}$ *OR Shortcut* $\dfrac{\overset{1}{\cancel{4}}}{\underset{3}{\cancel{12}}} = \dfrac{1}{3}$

14. $\dfrac{15}{18} = \dfrac{\overset{1}{\cancel{3}} \times 5}{\underset{1}{\cancel{3}} \times 6} = \dfrac{5}{6}$ *OR Shortcut* $\dfrac{\overset{5}{\cancel{15}}}{\underset{6}{\cancel{18}}} = \dfrac{5}{6}$

15. $\dfrac{6}{30} = \dfrac{\overset{1}{\cancel{2}} \times 3}{\underset{1}{\cancel{2}} \times 15} = \dfrac{3}{15} = \dfrac{1 \times \overset{1}{\cancel{3}}}{\underset{1}{\cancel{3}} \times 5} = \dfrac{1}{5}$ *OR Shortcut* $\dfrac{\overset{\overset{1}{\cancel{3}}}{\cancel{6}}}{\underset{\underset{5}{\cancel{15}}}{\cancel{30}}} = \dfrac{1}{5}$

16. $\dfrac{40}{100} = \dfrac{4 \times \overset{1}{\cancel{10}}}{10 \times \underset{1}{\cancel{10}}} = \dfrac{4}{10} = \dfrac{\overset{1}{\cancel{2}} \times 2}{\underset{1}{\cancel{2}} \times 5} = \dfrac{2}{5}$ *OR Shortcut* $\dfrac{\overset{\overset{2}{\cancel{4}}}{\cancel{40}}}{\underset{\underset{5}{\cancel{10}}}{\cancel{100}}} = \dfrac{2}{5}$

17. $\dfrac{1}{2} \quad \dfrac{2}{4}\overset{1}{\underset{2}{}}$
$\dfrac{1}{2} = \dfrac{1}{2}$
yes

18. $\dfrac{9}{11} \quad \dfrac{\overset{9}{\cancel{54}}}{\underset{11}{\cancel{66}}}$
$\dfrac{9}{11} = \dfrac{9}{11}$
yes

19. $\frac{2}{3}$ $\frac{\cancel{9}^{\,3}}{21_{\,7}}$

$\frac{2}{3} \neq \frac{3}{7}$

no

20. $\frac{7}{12}$ $\frac{\cancel{\cancel{28}}^{\;\;7}}{\cancel{60}}$ $\frac{^{\cancel{30}}}{15}$

$\frac{7}{12} \neq \frac{7}{15}$

no

2.2 Practice Multiplying Fractions

1. $\frac{3}{4} \times \frac{5}{11} = \frac{15}{44}$

2. $\frac{3}{5} \times \frac{4}{7} = \frac{12}{35}$

3. $\frac{\cancel{8}^{\,1}}{\cancel{9}_{\,1}} \times \frac{\cancel{27}^{\,3}}{\cancel{16}_{\,2}} = \frac{3}{2} = 1\frac{1}{2}$

4. $\frac{\cancel{8}^{\,1}}{\cancel{9}_{\,1}} \times \frac{\cancel{45}^{\,5}}{\cancel{56}_{\,7}} = \frac{5}{7}$

5. $\frac{\cancel{5}^{\,1}}{\cancel{24}_{\,4}^{\;8}} \times \frac{\cancel{18}^{\;\cancel{6}^{\;\cancel{3}^{\;1}}}}{\cancel{15}_{\,1}^{\;3}} = \frac{1}{4}$

6. $\frac{\cancel{12}^{\,4}}{17} \times \frac{\cancel{3}^{\,1}}{\cancel{27}_{\,9}_{\,3}} = \frac{4}{51}$

7. $\frac{2}{11} \times 4 = \frac{2}{11} \times \frac{4}{1} = \frac{8}{11}$

8. $9 \times \frac{7}{36} = \frac{\cancel{9}^{\,1}}{1} \times \frac{7}{\cancel{36}_{\,4}} = \frac{7}{4} = 1\frac{3}{4}$

9. $2\frac{3}{5} \times \frac{9}{11} = \frac{13}{5} \times \frac{9}{11} = \frac{117}{55} = 2\frac{7}{55}$

10. $4\frac{1}{3} \times 2\frac{2}{5} = \frac{13}{\cancel{3}_{\,1}} \times \frac{\cancel{12}^{\,4}}{5} = \frac{52}{5} = 10\frac{2}{5}$

11. $4\frac{3}{5} \times 1\frac{1}{5} = \frac{23}{5} \times \frac{6}{5} = \frac{138}{25} = 5\frac{13}{25}$

12. $3\frac{5}{6} \times 9 = \frac{23}{\cancel{6}_{\,2}} \times \frac{\cancel{9}^{\,3}}{1} = \frac{69}{2} = 34\frac{1}{2}$

13. $4\frac{2}{5} \times 14\frac{2}{9} = \frac{22}{5} \times \frac{128}{9} = \frac{2{,}816}{45} = 62\frac{26}{45}$

14. $5\dfrac{3}{4} \times 10\dfrac{5}{7} = \dfrac{23}{4} \times \dfrac{75}{7} = \dfrac{1,725}{28} = 61\dfrac{17}{28}$

15. $7\dfrac{3}{4} \times \dfrac{3}{7} = \dfrac{31}{4} \times \dfrac{3}{7} = \dfrac{93}{28} = 3\dfrac{9}{28}$

16. $5 \times 8\dfrac{3}{4} = \dfrac{5}{1} \times \dfrac{35}{4} = \dfrac{175}{4} = 43\dfrac{3}{4}$

17. $\dfrac{\overset{1}{\cancel{9}}}{\underset{1}{5}} \times \dfrac{\overset{1}{3}}{13} \times \dfrac{\overset{2}{\cancel{10}}}{\underset{\underset{1}{\cancel{3}}}{\cancel{27}}} = \dfrac{2}{13}$

18. $\dfrac{\overset{2}{\cancel{10}}}{\underset{1}{13}} \times \dfrac{\overset{2}{\cancel{26}}}{\underset{3}{\cancel{15}}} \times \dfrac{2}{3} = \dfrac{8}{9}$

19. $\dfrac{4}{5} \times \dfrac{15}{44} \times 4 = \dfrac{\overset{1}{\cancel{4}}}{\underset{1}{5}} \times \dfrac{\overset{3}{\cancel{15}}}{\underset{11}{\cancel{44}}} \times \dfrac{4}{1} = \dfrac{12}{11} = 1\dfrac{1}{11}$

20. $\dfrac{\overset{1}{\cancel{3}}}{\underset{1}{7}} \times \dfrac{\overset{2}{4}}{\underset{5}{10}} \times \dfrac{\overset{\overset{2}{\cancel{4}}}{\cancel{28}}}{\underset{\underset{3}{\cancel{6}}}{18}} = \dfrac{4}{15}$

2.3 Practice Dividing Fractions

1. $\dfrac{7}{10} \div \dfrac{14}{25} = \dfrac{\overset{1}{\cancel{7}}}{\underset{2}{\cancel{10}}} \times \dfrac{\overset{5}{\cancel{25}}}{\underset{2}{\cancel{14}}} = \dfrac{5}{4} = 1\dfrac{1}{4}$

2. $\dfrac{2}{5} \div \dfrac{5}{7} = \dfrac{2}{5} \times \dfrac{7}{5} = \dfrac{14}{25}$

3. $\dfrac{7}{8} \div \dfrac{2}{3} = \dfrac{7}{8} \times \dfrac{3}{2} = \dfrac{21}{16} = 1\dfrac{5}{16}$

4. $\dfrac{2}{9} \div \dfrac{1}{6} = \dfrac{2}{\underset{3}{\cancel{9}}} \times \dfrac{\overset{2}{\cancel{6}}}{1} = \dfrac{4}{3} = 1\dfrac{1}{3}$

5. $12 \div \dfrac{3}{4} = \dfrac{12}{1} \div \dfrac{3}{4} = \dfrac{\cancel{12}^{4}}{1} \times \dfrac{4}{\cancel{3}_{1}} = \dfrac{16}{1} = 16$

6. $\dfrac{5}{6} \div 18 = \dfrac{5}{6} \div \dfrac{18}{1} = \dfrac{5}{6} \times \dfrac{1}{18} = \dfrac{5}{108}$

7. $0 \div \dfrac{5}{16} = 0$

8. $1 \div \dfrac{3}{7} = \dfrac{1}{1} \times \dfrac{7}{3} = \dfrac{7}{3} = 2\dfrac{1}{3}$

9. $6\dfrac{3}{16} \div 1\dfrac{5}{8} = \dfrac{99}{16} \div \dfrac{13}{8} = \dfrac{99}{\cancel{16}_{2}} \times \dfrac{\cancel{8}^{1}}{13} = \dfrac{99}{26} = 3\dfrac{21}{26}$

10. $4\dfrac{2}{3} \div \dfrac{7}{27} = \dfrac{14}{3} \div \dfrac{7}{27} = \dfrac{\cancel{14}^{2}}{\cancel{3}_{1}} \times \dfrac{\cancel{27}^{9}}{\cancel{7}_{1}} = \dfrac{18}{1} = 18$

11. $6\dfrac{2}{5} \div 3 = \dfrac{32}{5} \div \dfrac{3}{1} = \dfrac{32}{5} \times \dfrac{1}{3} = \dfrac{32}{15} = 2\dfrac{2}{15}$

12. $2\dfrac{1}{3} \div 6\dfrac{5}{8} = \dfrac{7}{3} \div \dfrac{53}{8} = \dfrac{7}{3} \times \dfrac{8}{53} = \dfrac{56}{159}$

13. $2\dfrac{3}{8} \div 5\dfrac{3}{7} = \dfrac{19}{8} \div \dfrac{38}{7} = \dfrac{\cancel{19}^{1}}{8} \times \dfrac{7}{\cancel{38}_{2}} = \dfrac{7}{16}$

14. $\dfrac{24}{29} \div 0 =$ undefined or no solution

15. $2\dfrac{1}{15} \div 3\dfrac{1}{3} = \dfrac{31}{15} \div \dfrac{10}{3} = \dfrac{31}{\cancel{15}_{5}} \times \dfrac{\cancel{3}^{1}}{10} = \dfrac{31}{50}$

16. $6\dfrac{1}{2} \div 2\dfrac{3}{4} = \dfrac{13}{2} \div \dfrac{11}{4} = \dfrac{13}{\cancel{2}_{1}} \times \dfrac{\cancel{4}^{2}}{11} = \dfrac{26}{11} = 2\dfrac{4}{11}$

17. $12\dfrac{1}{2} \div 5\dfrac{5}{6} = \dfrac{25}{2} \div \dfrac{35}{6} = \dfrac{\cancel{25}^{5}}{\cancel{2}_{1}} \times \dfrac{\cancel{6}^{3}}{\cancel{35}_{7}} = \dfrac{15}{7} = 2\dfrac{1}{7}$

18. $4\frac{3}{5} \div 10 = \frac{23}{5} \div \frac{10}{1} = \frac{23}{5} \times \frac{1}{10} = \frac{23}{50}$

19. $6\frac{3}{4} \div 3\frac{1}{2} = \frac{27}{4} \div \frac{7}{2} = \frac{27}{\overset{}{\underset{2}{4}}} \times \frac{\overset{1}{2}}{7} = \frac{27}{14} = 1\frac{13}{14}$

20. $4\frac{5}{9} \div 2\frac{1}{3} = \frac{41}{9} \div \frac{7}{3} = \frac{41}{\overset{}{\underset{3}{9}}} \times \frac{\overset{1}{3}}{7} = \frac{41}{21} = 1\frac{20}{21}$

2.4 Practice Finding the Least Common Denominator (LCD)

1.
$$
\begin{array}{r|cc}
2 & 12 & 24 \\
2 & 6 & 12 \\
3 & 3 & 6 \\
\hline
& 1 & 2
\end{array}
$$
LCD = 2 • 2 • 3 • 1 • 2 = 24

2.
$$
\begin{array}{r|cc}
2 & 20 & 30 \\
5 & 10 & 15 \\
\hline
& 2 & 3
\end{array}
$$
LCD = 2 • 5 • 2 • 3 = 60

3.
$$
\begin{array}{r|cc}
2 & 40 & 10 \\
5 & 20 & 5 \\
\hline
& 4 & 1
\end{array}
$$
LCD = 2 • 5 • 4 • 1 = 40

4.
$$
\begin{array}{r|cc}
2 & 8 & 18 \\
\hline
& 4 & 9
\end{array}
$$
LCD = 2 • 4 • 9 = 72

5.
$$
\begin{array}{r|cc}
7 & 42 & 35 \\
\hline
& 6 & 5
\end{array}
$$
LCD = 7 • 6 • 5 = 210

6.
$$
\begin{array}{r|cc}
2 & 12 & 8 \\
2 & 6 & 4 \\
\hline
& 3 & 2
\end{array}
$$
LCD = 2 • 2 • 3 • 2 = 24

7.
$$
\begin{array}{r|cc}
5 & 40 & 25 \\
\hline
& 8 & 5
\end{array}
$$
LCD = 5 • 8 • 5 = 200

8. 2 | 40   50

   5 | 20   25

       4   5

LCD = 2 • 5 • 4 • 5 = 200

9. 2 | 32   40

   2 | 16   20

   2 | 8   10

       4   5

LCD = 2 • 2 • 2 • 4 • 5 = 160

10. 2 | 30   36

    3 | 15   18

        5   6

LCD = 2 • 3 • 5 • 6 = 180

11. 7 | 35   14

      5   2

LCD = 7 • 5 • 2 = 70

12. 11 | 33   22

       3   2

LCD = 11 • 3 • 2 = 66

13. 3 | 15   36

      5   12

LCD = 3 • 5 • 12 = 180

14. 3 | 21   9

      7   3

LCD = 3 • 7 • 3 = 63

15. 2 | 18   24

   3 | 9   12

       3   4

LCD = 2 • 3 • 3 • 4 = 72

16. 5 | 25   50

   5 | 5   10

       1   2

LCD = 5 • 5 • 1 • 2 = 50

17. 3 | 3   6   9

     1   2   3

LCD = 3 • 1 • 2 • 3 = 18

18.

$$3 \underline{)3 \quad 5 \quad 12}$$
$$1 \quad 5 \quad 4$$

LCD = 3 • 1 • 5 • 4 = 60

19.

$$2 \underline{)16 \quad 18 \quad 24}$$
$$2 \underline{)8 \quad 9 \quad 12}$$
$$2 \underline{)4 \quad 9 \quad 6}$$
$$3 \underline{)2 \quad 9 \quad 3}$$
$$2 \quad 3 \quad 1$$

LCD = 2 • 2 • 2 • 3 • 2 • 3 • 1 = 144

20.

$$2 \underline{)4 \quad 6 \quad 8}$$
$$2 \underline{)2 \quad 3 \quad 4}$$
$$1 \quad 3 \quad 2$$

LCD = 2 • 2 • 1 • 3 • 2 = 24

2.5 Practice Adding Fractions

1.

$$\begin{array}{r} \frac{1}{5} \\ + \frac{3}{5} \\ \hline \frac{4}{5} \end{array}$$

2.

$$7 \underline{)7 \quad 14}$$
$$1 \quad 2$$

LCD = 7 • 1 • 2 = 14

$$\frac{4}{7} • \frac{2}{2} = \frac{8}{14}$$
$$+ \frac{3}{14} = + \frac{3}{14}$$
$$\rule{2cm}{0.4pt}$$
$$\frac{11}{14}$$

3.

$$\underline{)11 \quad 5}$$

LCD = 11 • 5 = 55

$$\frac{9}{11} • \frac{5}{5} = \frac{45}{55}$$
$$+ \frac{4}{5} • \frac{11}{11} = + \frac{44}{55}$$
$$\rule{3cm}{0.4pt}$$
$$\frac{89}{55} = 1\frac{34}{55}$$

4.

$$\begin{array}{r} 7\frac{1}{8} \\ + 2\frac{5}{8} \\ \hline 9\frac{6}{8} = 9\frac{3}{4} \end{array}$$

5.

$5 \overline{)\, 5 \quad 10}$
$\phantom{5 \overline{)}} 1 \quad 2$

LCD = 5 • 1 • 2 = 10

$$5\frac{4}{5} \bullet \frac{2}{2} = \quad 5\frac{8}{10}$$

$$+\,3\frac{3}{10} \quad = \;+\; 3\frac{3}{10}$$

$$8\frac{11}{10}$$

$$8 + 1\frac{1}{10} = 9\frac{1}{10}$$

6.

$2 \overline{)\, 6 \quad 8}$
$\phantom{2 \overline{)}} 3 \quad 4$

LCD = 2 • 3 • 4 = 24

$$1\frac{5}{6} \bullet \frac{4}{4} = \quad 1\frac{20}{24}$$

$$+\,\frac{7}{8} \bullet \frac{3}{3} = \;+\; \frac{21}{24}$$

$$1\frac{41}{24}$$

$$1 + 1\frac{17}{24} = 2\frac{17}{24}$$

7.

$\overline{)\, 3 \quad 4}$

LCD = 3 • 4 = 12

$$4\frac{1}{3} \bullet \frac{4}{4} = \quad 4\frac{4}{12}$$

$$+\,2\frac{1}{4} \bullet \frac{3}{3} = \;+\; 2\frac{3}{12}$$

$$6\frac{7}{12}$$

8.

$2 \overline{)\, 10 \quad 8}$
$\phantom{2 \overline{)}} 5 \quad 4$

LCD = 2 • 5 • 4 = 40

$$47\frac{3}{10} \bullet \frac{4}{4} = \quad 47\frac{12}{40}$$

$$+\,26\frac{5}{8} \bullet \frac{5}{5} = \;+\; 26\frac{25}{40}$$

$$73\frac{37}{40}$$

9.

$5 \overline{)\, 20 \quad 15}$
$\phantom{5 \overline{)}} 4 \quad 3$

LCD = 5 • 4 • 3 = 60

$$34\frac{1}{20} \bullet \frac{3}{3} = \quad 34\frac{3}{60}$$

$$+\,45\frac{8}{15} \bullet \frac{4}{4} = \;+\; 45\frac{32}{60}$$

$$79\frac{35}{60} = 79\frac{7}{12}$$

10.

$7 \overline{)\, 14 \quad 7}$
$\phantom{7 \overline{)}} 2 \quad 1$

LCD = 7 • 2 • 1 = 14

$$25\frac{3}{14} \quad = \quad 25\frac{3}{14}$$

$$+\,58\frac{1}{7} \bullet \frac{2}{2} = \;+\; 58\frac{2}{14}$$

$$83\frac{5}{14}$$

11.

$11 \overline{)\, 33 \quad 11}$
$\phantom{11 \overline{)}} 3 \quad 1$

LCD = 11 • 3 • 1 = 33

$$2\frac{5}{33} \quad = \quad 2\frac{5}{33}$$

$$+\,\frac{3}{11} \bullet \frac{3}{3} = \;+\; \frac{9}{33}$$

$$2\frac{14}{33}$$

12.

$2 \overline{)\, 10 \quad 14}$
$\phantom{2 \overline{)}} 5 \quad 7$

LCD = 2 • 5 • 7 = 70

$$5\frac{3}{10} \bullet \frac{7}{7} = \quad 5\frac{21}{70}$$

$$+\,2\frac{1}{14} \bullet \frac{5}{5} = \;+\; 2\frac{5}{70}$$

$$7\frac{26}{70} = 7\frac{13}{35}$$

13.

$$\begin{array}{c|cc} & 9 & 4 \end{array}$$

LCD = $9 \cdot 4 = 36$

$$8\dfrac{2}{9} \cdot \dfrac{4}{4} = \quad 8\dfrac{8}{36}$$

$$+4\dfrac{3}{4} \cdot \dfrac{9}{9} = +4\dfrac{27}{36}$$

$$\overline{\qquad\qquad 12\dfrac{35}{36}}$$

14.

$$\begin{array}{c|cc} 2 & 6 & 10 \\ \hline & 3 & 5 \end{array}$$

LCD = $2 \cdot 3 \cdot 5 = 30$

$$4\dfrac{1}{6} \cdot \dfrac{5}{5} = \quad 4\dfrac{5}{30}$$

$$+13\dfrac{9}{10} \cdot \dfrac{3}{3} = +13\dfrac{27}{30}$$

$$\overline{\qquad\qquad 17\dfrac{32}{30}}$$

$$17 + 1\dfrac{1}{15} = 18\dfrac{1}{15}$$

15.

$$\begin{array}{c|cc} 3 & 9 & 15 \\ \hline & 3 & 5 \end{array}$$

LCD = $3 \cdot 3 \cdot 5 = 45$

$$6\dfrac{4}{9} \cdot \dfrac{5}{5} = \quad 6\dfrac{20}{45}$$

$$+12\dfrac{1}{15} \cdot \dfrac{3}{3} = +12\dfrac{3}{45}$$

$$\overline{\qquad\qquad 18\dfrac{23}{45}}$$

16.

$$\begin{array}{c|cc} & 5 & 8 \end{array}$$

LCD = $5 \cdot 8 = 40$

$$7\dfrac{3}{5} \cdot \dfrac{8}{8} = \quad 7\dfrac{24}{40}$$

$$+2\dfrac{1}{8} \cdot \dfrac{5}{5} = +2\dfrac{5}{40}$$

$$\overline{\qquad\qquad 9\dfrac{29}{40}}$$

17.

$$\begin{array}{c|ccc} 2 & 3 & 8 & 6 \\ 3 & 3 & 4 & 3 \\ \hline & 1 & 4 & 1 \end{array}$$

LCD = $2 \cdot 3 \cdot 1 \cdot 4 \cdot 1 = 24$

$$\dfrac{1}{3} \cdot \dfrac{8}{8} = \quad \dfrac{8}{24}$$

$$\dfrac{1}{8} \cdot \dfrac{3}{3} = \quad \dfrac{3}{24}$$

$$+\dfrac{1}{6} \cdot \dfrac{4}{4} = +\dfrac{4}{24}$$

$$\overline{\qquad\qquad \dfrac{15}{24} = \dfrac{5}{8}}$$

18.

$$\begin{array}{c|ccc} 2 & 12 & 14 & 21 \\ 3 & 6 & 7 & 21 \\ 7 & 2 & 7 & 7 \\ \hline & 2 & 1 & 1 \end{array}$$

LCD = $2 \cdot 3 \cdot 7 \cdot 2 \cdot 1 \cdot 1 = 84$

$$\dfrac{1}{12} \cdot \dfrac{7}{7} = \quad \dfrac{7}{84}$$

$$\dfrac{3}{14} \cdot \dfrac{6}{6} = \quad \dfrac{18}{84}$$

$$+\dfrac{4}{21} \cdot \dfrac{4}{4} = +\dfrac{16}{84}$$

$$\overline{\qquad\qquad \dfrac{41}{84}}$$

19.

$$
\begin{array}{c|ccc}
2 & 20 & 15 & 10 \\
5 & 10 & 15 & 5 \\
\hline
 & 2 & 3 & 1
\end{array}
$$

LCD = 2 • 5 • 2 • 3 • 1 = 60

$$3\frac{1}{20} \bullet \frac{3}{3} = \quad 3\frac{3}{60}$$

$$7\frac{1}{15} \bullet \frac{4}{4} = \quad 7\frac{4}{60}$$

$$+ 2\frac{3}{10} \bullet \frac{6}{6} = + 2\frac{18}{60}$$

$$\overline{\qquad\qquad 12\frac{25}{60} = 12\frac{5}{12}}$$

20.

$$
\begin{array}{c|ccc}
2 & 3 & 8 & 6 \\
3 & 3 & 4 & 3 \\
\hline
 & 1 & 4 & 1
\end{array}
$$

LCD = 2 • 3 • 1 • 4 • 1 = 24

$$27\frac{2}{3} \bullet \frac{8}{8} = \quad 27\frac{16}{24}$$

$$30\frac{5}{8} \bullet \frac{3}{3} = \quad 30\frac{15}{24}$$

$$+ 31\frac{5}{6} \bullet \frac{4}{4} = + 31\frac{20}{24}$$

$$\overline{\qquad\qquad 88\frac{51}{24}}$$

$$88 + 2\frac{1}{8} = 90\frac{1}{8}$$

2.6 Practice Subtracting Fractions

1.
$$\frac{3}{4}$$
$$-\frac{1}{4}$$
$$\overline{\frac{2}{4}} = \frac{1}{2}$$

2.
$$\frac{84}{89}$$
$$-\frac{32}{89}$$
$$\overline{\frac{52}{89}}$$

3.

$$
\begin{array}{c|cc}
5 & 20 & 5 \\
\hline
 & 4 & 1
\end{array}
$$

LCD = 5 • 4 • 1 = 20

$$\frac{37}{20} = \quad \frac{37}{20}$$

$$-\frac{4}{5} \bullet \frac{4}{4} = -\frac{16}{20}$$

$$\overline{\qquad\qquad \frac{21}{20} = 1\frac{1}{20}}$$

4.

$$
\begin{array}{c|cc}
 & 9 & 7
\end{array}
$$

LCD = 9 • 7 = 63

$$\frac{3}{9} \bullet \frac{7}{7} = \quad \frac{21}{63}$$

$$-\frac{1}{7} \bullet \frac{9}{9} = -\frac{9}{63}$$

$$\overline{\qquad\qquad \frac{12}{63} = \frac{4}{21}}$$

5.

$$
\begin{array}{c|cc}
5 & 50 & 25 \\
5 & 10 & 5 \\
\hline
 & 2 & 1
\end{array}
$$

LCD = 5 • 5 • 2 • 1 = 50

$$\frac{9}{50} = \quad \frac{9}{50}$$

$$-\frac{2}{25} \bullet \frac{2}{2} = -\frac{4}{50}$$

$$\overline{\qquad\qquad \frac{5}{50} = \frac{1}{10}}$$

6.

$$
\begin{array}{c|cc}
2 & 12 & 30 \\
3 & 6 & 15 \\
& 2 & 5
\end{array}
$$

LCD = 2 • 3 • 2 • 5 = 60

$$\dfrac{5}{12} \bullet \dfrac{5}{5} = \dfrac{25}{60}$$

$$-\dfrac{7}{30} \bullet \dfrac{2}{2} = -\dfrac{14}{60}$$

$$\dfrac{11}{60}$$

7.

$$\dfrac{11}{24}$$

$$-\dfrac{0}{4}$$

$$\dfrac{11}{24}$$

8.

$$7\dfrac{11}{12}$$

$$-3\dfrac{5}{12}$$

$$4\dfrac{6}{12} = 4\dfrac{1}{2}$$

9.

$$6\dfrac{7}{8}$$

$$-4\dfrac{3}{8}$$

$$2\dfrac{4}{8} = 2\dfrac{1}{2}$$

10.

$$
\begin{array}{c|cc}
2 & 6 & 4 \\
& 3 & 2
\end{array}
$$

LCD = 2 • 3 • 2 = 12

$$18\dfrac{5}{6} \bullet \dfrac{2}{2} = \quad 18\dfrac{10}{12}$$

$$-10\dfrac{1}{4} \bullet \dfrac{3}{3} = -10\dfrac{3}{12}$$

$$8\dfrac{7}{12}$$

11.

$$
\begin{array}{c|cc}
2 & 8 & 4 \\
2 & 4 & 2 \\
& 2 & 1
\end{array}
$$

LCD = 2 • 2 • 2 • 1 = 8

$$10\dfrac{3}{8} = \overset{9\frac{8}{8}}{\cancel{10}\dfrac{3}{8}} = 9\dfrac{11}{8}$$

$$-1\dfrac{3}{4} \bullet \dfrac{2}{2} = -1\dfrac{6}{8} = -1\dfrac{6}{8}$$

$$8\dfrac{5}{8}$$

12.

$$
\begin{array}{c|cc}
2 & 6 & 4 \\
& 3 & 2
\end{array}
$$

LCD = 2 • 3 • 2 = 12

$$18\dfrac{1}{6} \bullet \dfrac{2}{2} = \ 18\overset{7\frac{12}{12}}{\dfrac{2}{12}} = \ 17\dfrac{14}{12}$$

$$-10\dfrac{3}{4} \bullet \dfrac{3}{3} = -10\dfrac{9}{12} = -10\dfrac{9}{12}$$

$$7\dfrac{5}{12}$$

13.

$$
\begin{array}{c|cc}
3 & 9 & 6 \\
& 3 & 2
\end{array}
$$

LCD = 3 • 3 • 2 = 18

$$12\dfrac{4}{9} \bullet \dfrac{2}{2} = 12\overset{1\frac{18}{18}}{\dfrac{8}{18}} = \ 11\dfrac{26}{18}$$

$$-7\dfrac{5}{6} \bullet \dfrac{3}{3} = -7\dfrac{15}{18} = -7\dfrac{15}{18}$$

$$4\dfrac{11}{18}$$

14.

$$1 = \frac{7}{7}$$
$$-\frac{3}{7} = -\frac{3}{7}$$
$$\overline{\quad\quad\frac{4}{7}}$$

15.

$$30 = 29\frac{7}{7}$$
$$-15\frac{3}{7} = -15\frac{3}{7}$$
$$\overline{\quad\quad 14\frac{4}{7}}$$

16.

$$\begin{array}{c|cc} 5 & 20 & 15 \\ & 4 & 3 \end{array}$$

LCD = 5 ● 4 ● 3 = 60

$$34\frac{1}{20} \bullet \frac{3}{3} = 34\overset{3\frac{60}{60}}{\cancel{}}\frac{3}{60} = \overset{2\;13}{\cancel{3\,3}}\frac{63}{60}$$
$$-25\frac{8}{15} \bullet \frac{4}{4} = -25\frac{32}{60} = -25\frac{32}{60}$$
$$\overline{\quad\quad 8\frac{31}{60}}$$

17.

$$\begin{array}{c|cc} 3 & 3 & 6 \\ & 1 & 2 \end{array}$$

LCD = 3 ● 1 ● 2 = 6

$$19\frac{1}{3} \bullet \frac{2}{2} = 19\frac{2}{6} = \overset{8\frac{6}{6}}{18}\frac{8}{6}$$
$$-14\frac{5}{6} = -14\frac{5}{6} = -14\frac{5}{6}$$
$$\overline{\quad\quad 4\frac{3}{6} = 4\frac{1}{2}}$$

18.

$$\begin{array}{c|cc} 5 & 20 & 15 \\ & 4 & 3 \end{array}$$

LCD = 5 ● 4 ● 3 = 60

$$12\frac{3}{20} \bullet \frac{3}{3} = 12\overset{1\frac{60}{60}}{\cancel{}}\frac{9}{60} = 11\frac{69}{60}$$
$$-7\frac{7}{15} \bullet \frac{4}{4} = -7\frac{28}{60} = -7\frac{28}{60}$$
$$\overline{\quad\quad 4\frac{41}{60}}$$

19.

$$\begin{array}{c|cc} 2 & 10 & 8 \\ & 5 & 4 \end{array}$$

LCD = 2 ● 5 ● 4 = 40

$$47\frac{3}{10} \bullet \frac{4}{4} = 47\overset{6\frac{40}{40}}{\cancel{}}\frac{12}{40} = 46\frac{52}{40}$$
$$-25\frac{5}{8} \bullet \frac{5}{5} = -25\frac{25}{40} = -25\frac{25}{40}$$
$$\overline{\quad\quad 21\frac{27}{40}}$$

20.

$$\begin{array}{c|cc} 2 & 12 & 10 \\ & 6 & 5 \end{array}$$

LCD = 2 ● 6 ● 5 = 60

$$8\frac{5}{12} \bullet \frac{5}{5} = \overset{7\frac{60}{60}}{\cancel{8}}\frac{25}{60} = 7\frac{85}{60}$$
$$-5\frac{9}{10} \bullet \frac{6}{6} = -5\frac{54}{60} = -5\frac{54}{60}$$
$$\overline{\quad\quad 2\frac{31}{60}}$$

2.7 Chapter Test for Fractions

Section 2.1

1. $\dfrac{58}{5}$
$$5\overline{)58} = 11\tfrac{3}{5}$$
$$\begin{array}{r} 11\tfrac{3}{5} \\ 5\overline{)58} \\ \underline{-5} \\ 08 \\ \underline{-5} \\ 3 \end{array}$$

2. $\dfrac{23}{2}$
$$\begin{array}{r} 11\tfrac{1}{2} \\ 2\overline{)23} \\ \underline{-2} \\ 03 \\ \underline{-2} \\ 1 \end{array}$$

3. $\dfrac{75}{6}$
$$\begin{array}{r} 12\tfrac{3}{6} = 12\tfrac{1}{2} \\ 6\overline{)75} \\ \underline{-6} \\ 15 \\ \underline{-12} \\ 3 \end{array}$$

4. $4\dfrac{6}{13} = \dfrac{(4 \times 13)+6}{13} = \dfrac{58}{13}$
  $\overset{52}{}$

5. $7\dfrac{3}{8} = \dfrac{(7 \times 8) + 3}{8} = \dfrac{59}{8}$
  $\overset{56}{}$

Section 2.2

6. $\dfrac{\overset{1}{8}}{\underset{1}{9}} \times \dfrac{\overset{3}{\cancel{54}}\,{}^{6}}{\cancel{32}\,{}_{4}\,{}_{2}} = \dfrac{3}{2} = 1\tfrac{1}{2}$

7. $3\dfrac{4}{5} \times \dfrac{15}{4} = \dfrac{19}{\underset{1}{\cancel{5}}} \times \dfrac{\cancel{15}\,{}^{3}}{4} = \dfrac{57}{4} = 14\tfrac{1}{4}$

8. $6 \times 5\dfrac{7}{8} = \dfrac{\overset{3}{\cancel{6}}}{1} \times \dfrac{47}{\cancel{8}\,{}_{4}} = \dfrac{141}{4} = 35\tfrac{1}{4}$

9. $\dfrac{\overset{1}{3}}{\underset{1}{8}} \times \dfrac{\overset{1}{5}}{\cancel{6}\,{}_{\underset{1}{2}}} \times \dfrac{\overset{2}{\cancel{16}}\,{}^{1}}{\underset{1}{5}} = \dfrac{1}{1} = 1$

Section 2.3

10. $\dfrac{8}{15} \div \dfrac{4}{25} = \dfrac{\overset{2}{\cancel{8}}}{\underset{3}{\cancel{15}}} \times \dfrac{\overset{5}{\cancel{25}}}{\underset{1}{\cancel{4}}} = \dfrac{10}{3} = 3\dfrac{1}{3}$

11. $\dfrac{1}{2} \div 0 =$ undefined or no solution

12. $7\dfrac{7}{9} \div 3\dfrac{7}{21} = \dfrac{70}{9} \div \dfrac{70}{21} = \dfrac{\overset{1}{\cancel{70}}}{\underset{3}{\cancel{9}}} \times \dfrac{\overset{7}{\cancel{21}}}{\underset{1}{\cancel{70}}} = \dfrac{7}{3} = 2\dfrac{1}{3}$

Sections 2.4 and 2.5

13.
$$
\begin{array}{r}
\dfrac{1}{5} \\[4pt]
+\,\dfrac{4}{5} \\[4pt]
\hline
\dfrac{5}{5} = 1
\end{array}
$$

14. LCD $= 3 \bullet 4 = 12$ $\left|\underline{\begin{array}{cc} 3 & 4 \end{array}}\right.$

$$
\begin{array}{r}
4\dfrac{1}{3} \bullet \dfrac{4}{4} = \quad 4\dfrac{4}{12} \\[6pt]
+\,6\dfrac{3}{4} \bullet \dfrac{3}{3} = +\,6\dfrac{9}{12} \\[6pt]
\hline
10\dfrac{13}{12}
\end{array}
$$

$\dfrac{13}{12} = 1\dfrac{1}{12}$

$10 + 1\dfrac{1}{12} = 11\dfrac{1}{12}$

15. LCD $= 3 \bullet 1 \bullet 8 \bullet 3 = 72$

$3\big|\underline{\begin{array}{ccc} 3 & 8 & 9 \end{array}}$
  $\quad\; 1 \quad\; 8 \quad\; 3$

$$
\begin{array}{r}
\dfrac{1}{3} \bullet \dfrac{24}{24} = \dfrac{24}{72} \\[6pt]
\dfrac{1}{8} \bullet \dfrac{9}{9} = \dfrac{9}{72} \\[6pt]
+\,\dfrac{1}{9} \bullet \dfrac{8}{8} = \dfrac{8}{72} \\[6pt]
\hline
\dfrac{41}{72}
\end{array}
$$

16. LCD $= 2 \bullet 5 \bullet 2 \bullet 3 \bullet 1 = 60$

$2\big|\underline{\begin{array}{ccc} 20 & 15 & 10 \end{array}}$
$5\big|\underline{\begin{array}{ccc} 10 & 15 & 5 \end{array}}$
  $\quad\; 2 \quad\;\; 3 \quad\; 1$

$$
\begin{array}{r}
3\dfrac{3}{20} \bullet \dfrac{3}{3} = 3\dfrac{9}{60} \\[6pt]
7\dfrac{7}{15} \bullet \dfrac{4}{4} = 7\dfrac{28}{60} \\[6pt]
+\,2\dfrac{1}{10} \bullet \dfrac{6}{6} = 2\dfrac{6}{60} \\[6pt]
\hline
12\dfrac{43}{60}
\end{array}
$$

Sections 2.4 and 2.6

17. $\text{LCD} = 2 \bullet 3 \bullet 2 = 12$

$$2 \underline{)6 \qquad 4}$$
$$\qquad 3 \qquad 2$$

$$\frac{5}{6} \bullet \frac{2}{2} = \frac{10}{12}$$
$$-\frac{3}{4} \bullet \frac{3}{3} = -\frac{9}{12}$$
$$\frac{1}{12}$$

18. $\text{LCD} = 2 \bullet 3 \bullet 7 = 42$

$$2 \underline{)6 \qquad 14}$$
$$\qquad 3 \qquad 7$$

$$7\frac{5}{6} \bullet \frac{7}{7} = 7\frac{35}{42}$$
$$-4\frac{3}{14} \bullet \frac{3}{3} = -4\frac{9}{42}$$
$$3\frac{26}{42} = 3\frac{13}{21}$$

19. $4\frac{8}{8}$

$$\cancel{5}\frac{3}{8} = 4\frac{11}{8}$$
$$-2\frac{5}{8} = -2\frac{5}{8}$$
$$2\frac{6}{8} = 2\frac{3}{4}$$

20. $\text{LCD} = 2 \bullet 2 \bullet 2 \bullet 3 = 24$

$$2 \underline{)8 \qquad 12}$$
$$2 \underline{)4 \qquad 6}$$
$$\qquad 2 \qquad 3$$

$$5\frac{24}{24}$$
$$16\frac{1}{8} \bullet \frac{3}{3} = 1\cancel{6}\frac{3}{24} = 15\frac{27}{24}$$
$$-13\frac{11}{12} \bullet \frac{2}{2} = -13\frac{22}{24} = -13\frac{22}{24}$$
$$2\frac{5}{24}$$

3.0 **Pretest for Decimal Numbers**

Sections 3.1 and 3.2

1. 36.⑤9 = 36.6

Section 3.3

2. $\overset{1}{7.23}00$
    $+\ 5.9614$
    _____
    13.1914

3. $2\overset{4\ \overset{9}{\cancel{1}}\overset{10}{0}\ 0\ 10}{\cancel{5}.0\cancel{1}0}$
    $-\ 14.732$
    _____
    10.278

Section 3.4

4. $\overset{\overset{\overset{12}{13\ 1}}{25\ 1}}{53.72}$
    $\times\ 4.58$
    _____
    $\overset{2\ 2}{4\,29\,76}$
    $\overset{1}{26\,86\,0}$
    $2\,14\,88$
    _____
    $246.03\,76$

Section 3.5

5. $7.③5 = 7.4$

    $\overset{\overset{1}{1}}{51.2\,)\overline{376.4.\,2\,0}}$
    $\underline{-358\ 4}$
    $\quad 180\ 2$
    $\underline{-153\ 6}$
    $\qquad 26\ \ 6\ 0$
    $\underline{\ -25\ \ 6\ 0}$
    $\qquad\ \ 1\ \ 0\ 0$

Section 3.6

6. $\dfrac{\overset{1}{\cancel{5}}\ \cancel{125}}{\underset{8}{\cancel{40}}\ \cancel{1,000}} = \dfrac{1}{8}$

7.
$$
\begin{array}{r}
0.8 \\
5\overline{)4.0} \\
-4\ 0 \\
\hline
0
\end{array}
$$

Section 3.7

8. a.   0.0119
       0.0910
       0.0191
       0.0100

   b.   0.0100
       0.0119
       0.0191
       0.0910

   c.   0.01 0.0119 0.0191 0.091

9. a. $5\overline{)5\quad 15\quad 25}$
       $1\quad 3\quad 5$

   LCD = 5 • 1 • 3 • 5 = 75

   b. $\dfrac{1}{5} = \dfrac{15}{75}$

       $\dfrac{7}{15} = \dfrac{35}{75}$

       $\dfrac{8}{25} = \dfrac{24}{75}$

   c. $\dfrac{15}{75}\quad \dfrac{24}{75}\quad \dfrac{35}{75}$

   d. $\dfrac{1}{5}\quad \dfrac{8}{25}\quad \dfrac{7}{15}$

10. a. $\dfrac{3}{25} =$
$$
\begin{array}{r}
0.12 \\
25\overline{)3.00} \\
-2\ 5 \\
\hline
50 \\
-50 \\
\hline
0
\end{array}
$$

   b.   0.12 < 0.14

   c. $\dfrac{3}{25} < 0.14$

3.1 Practice Place Value

1. 4	5. 2	9. 8	13. 2	17. 3
2. 5	6. 6	10. 9	14. 1	18. 0
3. 7	7. 8	11. 5	15. 9	19. 6
4. 3	8. 3	12. 2	16. 8	20. 4

3.2 Practice Rounding Decimal Numbers

1. 33.④5 = **33.5**

2. ⑦4.561 = **70**

3. 234.3⑤7 = **234.36**

4. ②5 = **30**

5. 36.⑦58 = **36.8**

6. 345.⑥4 = **345.6**

7. 3④,785 = **35,000**

8. 7④.521 = **75**

9. 345.⑧56 = **345.9**

10. 2④.56 = **25**

11. ④56 = **500**

12. 24.276①4 = **24.2761**

13. 7⑥,476.23 = **76,000**

14. ⑤4 = **50**

15. 36.3③7 = **36.34**

16. ⑤64 = **600**

17. 1,362.27⑥3 = **1,362.276**

18. 3⑥.342 = **36**

19. 24,⑦76.25 = **24,800**

20. 3⑥,132 = **36,000**

3.3 Practice Adding and Subtracting Decimal Numbers

1.   55.7
     + 23.2
    78.9

2.   111 1
      718.98
     + 496.69
    1,215.67

3.   1 1
      1.806
     + 4.856
    6.662

4.   1 11
      9.365
     +5.796
    15.161

5.   1
     79.061
     + 5.72**0**
    84.781

6.   11
      813.7**0**
     + 629.86
    1,443.56

7.
$$\overset{1}{1.86}$$
$$+\,23.2\textbf{0}$$
$$\overline{\textbf{25.06}}$$

8.
$$\overset{11\ \ 1}{26.905}$$
$$+\,7{,}643.457$$
$$\overline{\textbf{7,670.362}}$$

9.
$$\overset{11}{6.543}$$
$$12.61\textbf{0}$$
$$+\,304.8\textbf{00}$$
$$\overline{\textbf{323.953}}$$

10.
$$\overset{21\ \ 1}{18.297}$$
$$\overset{1}{\ \ }7.6\textbf{00}$$
$$+\,199.83\textbf{0}$$
$$\overline{\textbf{225.727}}$$

11.
$$\overset{5\ \,10}{7\cancel{6}.0}$$
$$-\,4.8$$
$$\overline{\textbf{7 1.2}}$$

12.
$$\overset{7\,11}{\underset{}{\overset{1\ \ \ 12}{\overset{\ \ \ \ 2\,10}{8\cancel{2}.\cancel{3}\,0}}}}$$
$$-\,4 3.9 4$$
$$\overline{\textbf{3 8.3 6}}$$

13.
$$\overset{7\,14}{\underset{}{\overset{4\ \ 14}{1\cancel{8}\cancel{5}.47}}}$$
$$-\,6 7.5\textbf{0}$$
$$\overline{\textbf{1 1 7.97}}$$

14.
$$\overset{1\ 13}{\underset{}{\overset{3\,13}{\overset{\ \ \ 7\,10}{2\cancel{4}3.9\cancel{8}\textbf{0}}}}}$$
$$-\,8 4.2 5 6$$
$$\overline{\textbf{1 5 9.7 2 4}}$$

15.
$$4{,}986.25$$
$$-\,3{,}615.24$$
$$\overline{\textbf{1,371.01}}$$

16.
$$\overset{9\,10}{\underset{}{\overset{9\cancel{10}}{\overset{1\ \cancel{10}}{1\cancel{2}.000}}}}$$
$$-\,1.263$$
$$\overline{\textbf{10.737}}$$

17.
$$\overset{9\,10}{\underset{}{\overset{9\,\cancel{10}}{\overset{4\ \cancel{10}}{1.\cancel{5}\,0\,0\,0\,0}}}}$$
$$-\,0.0 3 7 5 2$$
$$\overline{\textbf{1.4 6 2 4 8}}$$

18.
$$25.754$$
$$-\,25.752$$
$$\overline{\textbf{0.002}}$$

19.
$$\overset{4\ 13}{\underset{}{\overset{9\,10}{\overset{3\,\cancel{10}}{17.\cancel{5}\cancel{4}\,0\,0}}}}$$
$$-\,2.0 4 3 2$$
$$\overline{\textbf{1 5.4 9 6 8}}$$

20.
$$\overset{9\,12}{\underset{}{\overset{9\,\cancel{10}}{\overset{0\,1\,\cancel{0}}{1\cancel{0}0.232}}}}$$
$$-\,0.4\textbf{00}$$
$$\overline{\textbf{99.832}}$$

3.4 Practice Multiplying Decimal Numbers

1.
$$0.6$$
$$\times\,0.9$$
$$\overline{\textbf{0.54}}$$

2.
$$\overset{1}{0.13}$$
$$\times\,0.5$$
$$\overline{\textbf{0.065}}$$

3.
$$\overset{2\,6}{\underset{}{\overset{2\,7}{0.028}}}$$
$$\times\,0.89$$
$$\overline{\textbf{252}}$$
$$\underline{\textbf{224}}$$
$$\textbf{0.02492}$$

4.
$$\overset{1\,2}{\underset{}{\overset{2\,5}{0.0437}}}$$
$$\times\,0.48$$
$$\overset{1}{\underline{\textbf{1\,3496}}}$$
$$\underline{\textbf{1748}}$$
$$\textbf{0.020976}$$

5.
$$\overset{1\ 1\ 2}{6.2\,34}$$
$$\times\,2.25$$
$$\overset{1\,1\,1}{\underline{\textbf{1\,31170}}}$$
$$\textbf{12468}$$
$$\underline{\textbf{12468}}$$
$$\textbf{14.026\,50} =$$
$$\textbf{14.0265}$$

6.
$$\overset{1\,2}{\underset{}{\overset{1\,2\,4}{\overset{1\,2\,5}{81.26}}}}$$
$$\times\,4.89$$
$$\overset{1}{\underline{\textbf{1\,73134}}}$$
$$\textbf{65\,008}$$
$$\underline{\textbf{325\,04}}$$
$$\textbf{397.36\,14}$$

7.
$$
\begin{array}{r}
232 \\
121 \\
11 \\
924.3 \\
\times\ 96.4 \\
\hline
221 \\
1\,3697\,2 \\
5\,5458 \\
83\,187 \\
\hline
89{,}102.5\,2
\end{array}
$$

8.
$$
\begin{array}{r}
1\ \ 1 \\
5\ \ 4 \\
5\ \ 4 \\
9.6501 \\
\times\ 129.8 \\
\hline
1 \\
{}_2 7\,72008 \\
2\,868509 \\
193\,002 \\
965\,01 \\
\hline
1{,}252.58298
\end{array}
$$

9.
$$
\begin{array}{r}
4\ \ 3 \\
19.07 \\
\times\ 0.05 \\
\hline
0.9535
\end{array}
$$

10.
$$
\begin{array}{r}
1\,66 \\
5{,}167 \\
\times\ 0.19 \\
\hline
1 \\
465\,03 \\
516\,7 \\
\hline
981.73
\end{array}
$$

11.
$$
\begin{array}{r}
1\,52 \\
2.163 \\
\times\ 0.008 \\
\hline
0.017304
\end{array}
$$

12.
$$
\begin{array}{r}
3\,3\ \ 4 \\
2\,2\ \ 3 \\
0.6718 \\
\times\ 50.04 \\
\hline
1\,26872 \\
33\,59000\,0 \\
\hline
33.616872
\end{array}
$$

13.
$$
\begin{array}{r}
1 \\
13 \\
12\,6 \\
\times\ 3.5 \\
\hline
1 \\
1\,630 \\
378 \\
\hline
441.0 = 441
\end{array}
$$

14.
$$
\begin{array}{r}
5 \\
3 \\
4 \\
5{,}060 \\
\times\ 9.57 \\
\hline
1 \\
1\,354\,20 \\
2530\,0 \\
45540 \\
\hline
48{,}424.20 = \\
48{,}424.2
\end{array}
$$

15.
$$
\begin{array}{r}
6 \\
3 \\
7{,}090 \\
\times\ 1.74 \\
\hline
2 \\
1\,28360 \\
49630 \\
7090 \\
\hline
12{,}336.60 = \\
12{,}336.6
\end{array}
$$

16.
$$
\begin{array}{r}
4 \\
0.06 \\
\times\ 0.07 \\
\hline
0.0042
\end{array}
$$

17.
$$
\begin{array}{r}
4\ \ 1 \\
70.92 \\
\times\ 2.05 \\
\hline
1 \\
3\,5460 \\
141\,840 \\
\hline
145.38\,60 = \\
145.386
\end{array}
$$

18.
$$
\begin{array}{r}
5\ \ 2 \\
5\ \ 2 \\
8.703 \\
\times\ 8.08 \\
\hline
11 \\
1\,1\,69624 \\
69\,6240 \\
\hline
70.32024
\end{array}
$$

19.
$$
\begin{array}{r}
6{,}523.7 \\
\times\ 0.001 \\
\hline
6.5237
\end{array}
$$

20.
$$
\begin{array}{r}
3\,4 \\
0.0056 \\
\times\ 0.07 \\
\hline
0.000392
\end{array}
$$

3.5 Practice Dividing Decimal Numbers

1.
$$4\overline{)0.044}$$
quotient: 0.011
$$
\begin{array}{r}
-4 \\
\hline
04 \\
-4 \\
\hline
0
\end{array}
$$

2.
$$5\overline{)0.01290}$$
quotient: 0.00258
$$
\begin{array}{r}
-10 \\
\hline
29 \\
-25 \\
\hline
40 \\
-40 \\
\hline
0
\end{array}
$$

3.
$$64\overline{)3.6160}$$
quotient: 0.0565   (carries: 2 2 2)
$$
\begin{array}{r}
-3\,20 \\
\hline
416 \\
-384 \\
\hline
320 \\
-320 \\
\hline
0
\end{array}
$$

4.
$$0.5\overline{)32.1.5}$$
quotient: 64.3
$$
\begin{array}{r}
-30 \\
\hline
2\,1 \\
-2\,0 \\
\hline
1\,5 \\
-15 \\
\hline
0
\end{array}
$$

5.
$$12.2\overline{)9.7.6}$$
quotient: 0.8   (11)
$$
\begin{array}{r}
-9\,7\,6 \\
\hline
0
\end{array}
$$

6.
$$0.85\overline{)41.90.5}$$
quotient: 49.3   (carries: 1 4 2)
$$
\begin{array}{r}
-34\,0 \\
\hline
7\,90 \\
-7\,65 \\
\hline
25\,5 \\
-25\,5 \\
\hline
0
\end{array}
$$

7.
$$1.87\overline{)170.65.62}$$
quotient: 91.26   (carries: 5 4 / 1 1 / 7 6)
$$
\begin{array}{r}
-168\,3 \\
\hline
2\,35 \\
-187 \\
\hline
486 \\
-374 \\
\hline
1122 \\
-1122 \\
\hline
0
\end{array}
$$

8.
$$0.69\overline{)8.44.974}$$
quotient: 12.246   (carries: 5 3 1 1)
$$
\begin{array}{r}
-6\,9 \\
\hline
1\,54 \\
-1\,38 \\
\hline
169 \\
-138 \\
\hline
317 \\
-276 \\
\hline
4\,14 \\
-414 \\
\hline
0
\end{array}
$$

9.
$$0.07\overline{)0.81.13}$$
quotient: 11.59
$$
\begin{array}{r}
-7 \\
\hline
11 \\
-7 \\
\hline
4\,1 \\
-3\,5 \\
\hline
63 \\
-63 \\
\hline
0
\end{array}
$$

10.
$$0.31\overline{)40.30.}$$
quotient: 1 30. = 130
$$
\begin{array}{r}
-31 \\
\hline
9\,3 \\
-9\,3 \\
\hline
00
\end{array}
$$

11.
$$0.28\overline{)95.20.}$$
quotient: 3 40. = 340   (carries: 3 2)
$$
\begin{array}{r}
-84 \\
\hline
11\,2 \\
-112 \\
\hline
00
\end{array}
$$

12.
$$3.6\overline{)75.6.}$$
quotient: 2 1. = 21   (carry: 1)
$$
\begin{array}{r}
-72 \\
\hline
3\,6 \\
-3\,6 \\
\hline
0
\end{array}
$$

13.

$$\overset{2}{\underset{2}{1}}$$

$$2\,835.\boxed{9}\,1 \overset{\Downarrow}{=} 2{,}835.9$$

$$0.023\overline{)65.226.\,0\,0}$$

```
    -46
    ‿‿‿    ‿‿‿
     19 2
    -18 4
      82
     -69
      136
     -115
       21 0
      -20 7
         30
        -2 3
          7
```

14.

$$\overset{3}{}$$

$$0.\boxed{0}\,7 \overset{\Downarrow}{=} 0.1$$

$$7.05\overline{)0.49.\,7\,7}$$

```
     ‿‿
    -49 3 5
       4 2
```

15.

$$\overset{2\,2\,.}{\underset{1\,1}{\overset{1\,1}{}}}$$

$$56.\boxed{3}\,9 = 56.4$$

$$1.33\overline{)75.00.\,0\,0}$$

```
    ‿‿     ‿‿
    -66 5
     8 50
    -7 98
      52 0
     -39 9
      12 10
     -11 97
       13
```

16.

$$\overset{1}{\underset{1}{}}$$

$$0.2\boxed{2}\,0 \overset{\Downarrow}{=} 0.22$$

$$26\overline{)5.7\,2\,9}$$

```
    -52
     5 2
    -5 2
      0 9
```

17.

$$\overset{1\,4}{\underset{1\,6}{\overset{1\,6}{}}}$$

$$1.8\boxed{8}\,6 \overset{\Downarrow}{=} 1.89$$

$$3.181\overline{)6.000.0\,00}$$

```
    ‿‿‿‿     ‿‿‿
    -3 181
     2 8190
    -2 5448
      274 2 0
     -25 44 8
       197 2 0
      -190 86
         6 3 4
```

18.

$$12.1\boxed{2}\,3 \overset{\Downarrow}{=} 12.12$$

$$1.23\overline{)14.91.1\,2\,9}$$

```
    -12 3
      2 61
     -2 46
       15 1
      -12 3
        2 82
       -2 46
         3 6 9
        -3 6 9
           0
```

19.

$$\begin{array}{r} \overset{1}{5}\overset{2}{6} \\ 2.57\overline{)\,0.49.61\;00} \end{array}$$

$0.19\,\textcircled{3}\,0 = 0.193$

$$\begin{array}{r} -25\,7 \\ \hline 23\,91 \\ -23\,13 \\ \hline 78\,0 \\ -77\,1 \\ \hline 9\,0 \\ -0 \\ \hline 9\,0 \end{array}$$

20.

$$\begin{array}{r} \overset{1}{\overset{1}{\overset{1}{2}}}2 \\ 0.23\overline{)\,45.57.60\;00} \end{array}$$

$198.15\,\textcircled{6}\,5 = 198.157$

$$\begin{array}{r} -23 \\ \hline 225 \\ -207 \\ \hline 187 \\ -184 \\ \hline 36 \\ -23 \\ \hline 130 \\ -115 \\ \hline 15\,0 \\ -13\,8 \\ \hline 1\,2\,0 \\ -1\,15 \\ \hline 5 \end{array}$$

3.6 Practice Converting Decimals and Fractions

1. $\dfrac{\cancel{25}^{\,1}}{\cancel{100}_{\,4}} = \dfrac{1}{4}$

2. $17\dfrac{7}{10}$

3. $\dfrac{\cancel{375}^{\,3}}{\cancel{1000}_{\,8}} = \dfrac{3}{8}$

4. $\dfrac{\cancel{2}^{\,1}}{\cancel{10}_{\,5}} = \dfrac{1}{5}$

5. $865\dfrac{\cancel{75}^{\,3}}{\cancel{100}_{\,4}} = 865\dfrac{3}{4}$

6. $\dfrac{\cancel{625}^{\,5}}{\cancel{1000}_{\,8}} = \dfrac{5}{8}$

7. $34\dfrac{\cancel{5}^{\,1}}{\cancel{10}_{\,2}} = 34\dfrac{1}{2}$

8. $\dfrac{\cancel{35}^{\,7}}{\cancel{100}_{\,20}} = \dfrac{7}{20}$

9. $5\dfrac{9}{100}$

10. $\dfrac{\cancel{75}^{\,3}}{\cancel{1000}_{\,40}} = \dfrac{3}{40}$

11. $\begin{array}{r} 0.8 \\ 5\overline{)\,4.0} \\ -4\,0 \\ \hline 0 \end{array}$

12. $\begin{array}{r} 0.33 = 0.\overline{3} \\ 3\overline{)\,1.00} \\ -9 \\ \hline 10 \\ -9 \\ \hline 1 \end{array}$

$$\begin{array}{r} 0.625 \\ 8\overline{)5.000} \\ -48 \\ \hline 20 \\ -16 \\ \hline 40 \\ -40 \\ \hline 0 \end{array}$$
13.

$$\begin{array}{r} 0.2 \\ 5\overline{)1.0} \\ -10 \\ \hline 0 \end{array}$$
14.

$$\begin{array}{r} 0.25 \\ 4\overline{)1.00} \\ -8 \\ \hline 20 \\ -20 \\ \hline 0 \end{array}$$
15.

$$\begin{array}{r} 0.75 \\ 4\overline{)3.00} \\ -28 \\ \hline 20 \\ -20 \\ \hline 0 \end{array}$$
16.

$$\begin{array}{r} 0.35 \\ 20\overline{)7.00} \\ -6\,0 \\ \hline 1\,00 \\ -1\,00 \\ \hline 0 \end{array}$$
17.

$$\begin{array}{r} 3 \quad 0.36 \\ 1 \\ 25\overline{)9.00} \\ -7\,5 \\ \hline 1\,50 \\ -1\,50 \\ \hline 0 \end{array}$$
18.

$$\begin{array}{r} 0.4 \\ 5\overline{)2.0} \\ -2\,0 \\ \hline 0 \end{array}$$
19.

$$\begin{array}{r} 0.375 \\ 8\overline{)3.000} \\ -2\,4 \\ \hline 60 \\ -56 \\ \hline 40 \\ -40 \\ \hline 0 \end{array}$$
20.

3.7 Comparing Decimal Numbers and Fractions

1. a. 0.2630
   0.2632
   0.2600
   0.2000
   b. 0.2000
   0.2600
   0.2630
   0.2632
   c. 0.2 0.26 0.263 0.2632

2. a. 0.4730
   0.4720
   0.4000
   0.4732
   b. 0.4000
   0.4720
   0.4730
   0.4732
   c. 0.4 0.472 0.473 0.4732

3. a. 0.07400
   0.07421
   0.07440
   0.07240
   b. 0.07240
   0.07400
   0.07421
   0.07440
   c. 0.0724 0.074 0.07421 0.0744

4. a. 0.26262
   0.62620
   0.62000
   0.26200
   b. 0.26200
   0.26262
   0.62000
   0.62620
   c. 0.262 0.26262 0.62 0.6262

5. a. 0.240
   0.210
   0.401
   0.241
   b. 0.210
   0.240
   0.241
   0.401
   c. 0.21 0.24 0.241 0.401

6. a. 0.0426
   0.4000
   0.0461
   0.0600
   b. 0.0426
   0.0461
   0.0600
   0.4000
   c. 0.0426 0.0461 0.06 0.4

7. a.

2	3	2	6
3	3	1	3
	1	1	1

LCD = 2 • 3 • 1 • 1 • 1 = 6

b. $\dfrac{2}{3} = \dfrac{4}{6}$

$\dfrac{1}{2} = \dfrac{3}{6}$

$\dfrac{5}{6} = \dfrac{5}{6}$

c. $\dfrac{3}{6}\ \ \dfrac{4}{6}\ \ \dfrac{5}{6}$

d. $\dfrac{1}{2}\ \ \dfrac{2}{3}\ \ \dfrac{5}{6}$

8. a.

2	24	15	30
3	12	15	15
5	4	5	5
	4	1	1

LCD = 2 • 3 • 5 • 4 • 1 • 1 = 120

b. $\dfrac{5}{24} = \dfrac{25}{120}$

$\dfrac{11}{15} = \dfrac{88}{120}$

$\dfrac{7}{30} = \dfrac{28}{120}$

c. $\dfrac{25}{120}\ \ \dfrac{28}{120}\ \ \dfrac{88}{120}$

d. $\dfrac{5}{24}\ \ \dfrac{7}{30}\ \ \dfrac{11}{15}$

9. a.

$3 \overline{)\begin{array}{ccc} 12 & 21 & 3 \end{array}}$
$\phantom{3 \overline{)}} \begin{array}{ccc} 4 & 7 & 1 \end{array}$

LCD = 3 • 4 • 7 • 1 = 84

b. $\dfrac{7}{12} = \dfrac{49}{84}$

$\dfrac{1}{21} = \dfrac{4}{84}$

$\dfrac{2}{3} = \dfrac{56}{84}$

c. $\dfrac{4}{84} \quad \dfrac{49}{84} \quad \dfrac{56}{84}$

d. $\dfrac{1}{21} \quad \dfrac{7}{12} \quad \dfrac{2}{3}$

10. a.

$2 \overline{)\begin{array}{ccc} 16 & 18 & 24 \end{array}}$
$2 \overline{)\begin{array}{ccc} 8 & 9 & 12 \end{array}}$
$2 \overline{)\begin{array}{ccc} 4 & 9 & 6 \end{array}}$
$3 \overline{)\begin{array}{ccc} 2 & 9 & 3 \end{array}}$
$\phantom{3 \overline{)}}\begin{array}{ccc} 2 & 3 & 1 \end{array}$

LCD = 2 • 2 • 2 • 3 • 2 • 3 • 1 = 144

b. $\dfrac{5}{16} = \dfrac{45}{144}$

$\dfrac{11}{18} = \dfrac{88}{144}$

$\dfrac{1}{24} = \dfrac{6}{144}$

c. $\dfrac{6}{144} \quad \dfrac{45}{144} \quad \dfrac{88}{144}$

d. $\dfrac{1}{24} \quad \dfrac{5}{16} \quad \dfrac{11}{18}$

11. a.

$2 \overline{)\begin{array}{ccc} 15 & 12 & 8 \end{array}}$
$2 \overline{)\begin{array}{ccc} 15 & 6 & 4 \end{array}}$
$3 \overline{)\begin{array}{ccc} 15 & 3 & 2 \end{array}}$
$\phantom{3 \overline{)}}\begin{array}{ccc} 5 & 1 & 2 \end{array}$

LCD = 2 • 2 • 3 • 5 • 1 • 2 = 120

b. $\dfrac{7}{15} = \dfrac{56}{120}$

$\dfrac{11}{12} = \dfrac{110}{120}$

$\dfrac{7}{8} = \dfrac{105}{120}$

c. $\dfrac{56}{120} \quad \dfrac{105}{120} \quad \dfrac{110}{120}$

d. $\dfrac{7}{15} \quad \dfrac{7}{8} \quad \dfrac{11}{12}$

12. a.

$2 \overline{)\begin{array}{ccc} 8 & 4 & 16 \end{array}}$
$2 \overline{)\begin{array}{ccc} 4 & 2 & 8 \end{array}}$
$2 \overline{)\begin{array}{ccc} 2 & 1 & 4 \end{array}}$
$\phantom{2 \overline{)}}\begin{array}{ccc} 1 & 1 & 2 \end{array}$

LCD = 2 • 2 • 2 • 1 • 1 • 2 = 16

b. $\dfrac{1}{8} = \dfrac{2}{16}$

$\dfrac{3}{4} = \dfrac{12}{16}$

$\dfrac{9}{16} = \dfrac{9}{16}$

c. $\dfrac{2}{16} \quad \dfrac{9}{16} \quad \dfrac{12}{16}$

d. $\dfrac{1}{8} \quad \dfrac{9}{16} \quad \dfrac{3}{4}$

13. a.

$$\begin{array}{c|ccc} 5 & 5 & 4 & 15 \\ \hline & 1 & 4 & 3 \end{array}$$

LCD = 5 • 1 • 4 • 3 = 60

b. $\dfrac{2}{5} = \dfrac{24}{60}$

$\dfrac{1}{4} = \dfrac{15}{60}$

$\dfrac{7}{15} = \dfrac{28}{60}$

c. $\dfrac{15}{60} \quad \dfrac{24}{60} \quad \dfrac{28}{60}$

d. $\dfrac{1}{4} \quad \dfrac{2}{5} \quad \dfrac{7}{15}$

14. a. $\dfrac{5}{8} = $

$$\begin{array}{r} 0.625 \\ 8\overline{)5.000} \\ -48 \\ \hline 20 \\ -16 \\ \hline 40 \\ -40 \\ \hline 0 \end{array}$$

b. 0.627 > 0.625

c. 0.627 > $\dfrac{5}{8}$

15. a. $\dfrac{1}{4} = $

$$\begin{array}{r} 0.25 \\ 4\overline{)1.00} \\ -8 \\ \hline 20 \\ -20 \\ \hline 0 \end{array}$$

b. 0.30 > 0.25

c. 0.3 > $\dfrac{1}{4}$

16. a. $\dfrac{7}{20} = $

$$\begin{array}{r} 0.35 \\ 20\overline{)7.00} \\ -60 \\ \hline 100 \\ -100 \\ \hline 0 \end{array}$$

b. 0.35 < 0.36

c. $\dfrac{7}{20}$ < 0.36

17. a. $\dfrac{19}{40} = $

$$\begin{array}{r} 0.475 \\ 40\overline{)19.000} \\ -16\,0 \\ \hline 3\,00 \\ -2\,80 \\ \hline 200 \\ -200 \\ \hline 0 \end{array}$$

b. 0.475 > 0.470

c. $\dfrac{19}{40}$ > 0.47

18. a. $\dfrac{3}{4} = $

$$\begin{array}{r} 0.75 \\ 4\overline{)3.00} \\ -28 \\ \hline 20 \\ -20 \\ \hline 0 \end{array}$$

b. 0.75 = 0.75

c. $\dfrac{3}{4}$ = 0.75

19. a. $\dfrac{3}{5} = $

$$\begin{array}{r} 0.6 \\ 5\overline{)3.0} \\ -30 \\ \hline 0 \end{array}$$

b. 0.60 > 0.56

c. $\dfrac{3}{5}$ > 0.56

20. a. $\dfrac{7}{25} = $

$$\begin{array}{r} 0.28 \\ 25\overline{)7.00} \\ -50 \\ \hline 2\,00 \\ -2\,00 \\ \hline 0 \end{array}$$

b. 0.28 = 0.28

c. 0.28 = $\dfrac{7}{25}$

3.8 Chapter Test for Decimal Numbers

Section 3.1

1. 6   2. 4

Sections 3.1 and 3.2

3. 3.4⑤1 = 3.45   4. 57.⑧5 = 57.9

Section 3.3

5.   4.56
   + 2.30

    6.86

6.   12 1
     1.942
     0.230
   + 67.897

    70.069

7.   6 11
          115
      56⁷.²5⁹0   810
    - 4 3.8 7 1 5
    ----
    5 2 3.3 8 7 5

8.   6 12
           9 10
        2 ⁹10
      ⁷⁷.0 0 0
    - 7.5 9 6
    ----
     6 5.4 0 4

Section 3.4

9.   6 4
      3 2
      67.5
    × 0.84
    ----
     2 700
    54 00

    56.700 = 56.7

10.   4 2
      0.0063
    × 0.07

    0.000441

Section 3.5

11.   1 4
         1 5   6.5
    7.29)47.38.5
         -43 74
         ------
          364 5
         -364 5

              0

12.   1
        3 3   51.⑦2 = 51.7
        2 2
    1.45)75.00.00
         -72 5
         ------
          2 50
         -1 45

          1050
         -1015

           350
          -290

            60

Section 3.6

13.   ³⁶   3
      -- = -
     ₅10   5

14.   0.625
     8)5.000
      -48

        20
       -16

        40
       -40

         0

Section 3.7

15. a. 0.0893
   0.9000
   0.0839
   0.8900

   b. 0.0839
   0.0893
   0.8900
   0.9000

   c. 0.0839   0.0893   0.89   0.9

16. a. 1.525
   1.510
   1.526
   1.540

   b. 1.510
   1.525
   1.526
   1.540

   c. 1.51   1.525   1.526   1.54

17. a.

$$\begin{array}{r|rrr}
2 & 9 & 4 & 18 \\
3 & 9 & 2 & 9 \\
3 & 3 & 2 & 3 \\
  & 1 & 2 & 1
\end{array}$$

LCD = 2 • 3 • 3 • 1 • 2 • 1 = 36

   b. $\dfrac{5}{9} = \dfrac{20}{36}$

   $\dfrac{3}{4} = \dfrac{27}{36}$

   $\dfrac{11}{18} = \dfrac{22}{36}$

   c. $\dfrac{20}{36} \quad \dfrac{22}{36} \quad \dfrac{27}{36}$

   d. $\dfrac{5}{9} \quad \dfrac{11}{18} \quad \dfrac{3}{4}$

18. a.

$$\begin{array}{r|rrr}
7 & 7 & 21 & 35 \\
  & 1 & 3 & 5
\end{array}$$

LCD = 7 • 1 • 3 • 5 = 105

   b. $\dfrac{3}{7} = \dfrac{45}{105}$

   $\dfrac{4}{21} = \dfrac{20}{105}$

   $\dfrac{16}{35} = \dfrac{48}{105}$

   c. $\dfrac{20}{105} \quad \dfrac{45}{105} \quad \dfrac{48}{105}$

   d. $\dfrac{4}{21} \quad \dfrac{3}{7} \quad \dfrac{16}{35}$

19. a. $\dfrac{11}{50} =$

$$\begin{array}{r}
0.22 \\
50\overline{)11.00} \\
\underline{-10\,0} \\
1\,00 \\
\underline{-1\,00} \\
0
\end{array}$$

   b. 0.23 > 0.22

   c. 0.23 > $\dfrac{11}{50}$

20. a. $\dfrac{7}{10} =$

$$\begin{array}{r}
0.7 \\
10\overline{)7.0} \\
\underline{-7\,0} \\
0
\end{array}$$

   b. 0.69 < 0.70

   c. 0.69 < $\dfrac{7}{10}$

4.0 **Pretest for Percents, Ratios, and Proportions**

Section 4.1

1. $\dfrac{8}{3} = \dfrac{x}{15}$

$$\dfrac{\overset{1}{\cancel{3}}x}{\underset{1}{\cancel{3}}} = \dfrac{\overset{40}{\cancel{120}}}{\underset{1}{\cancel{3}}}$$

$x = 40$

Section 4.2

2. $\dfrac{x}{50} = \dfrac{5}{100}$

$$\dfrac{\overset{1}{\cancel{100}}x}{\underset{1}{\cancel{100}}} = \dfrac{250}{100}$$

$x = 2.5$

$$\begin{array}{r} 2.5 \\ 100\overline{)250.0} \\ -200 \\ \hline 50\ 0 \\ -50\ 0 \\ \hline 0 \end{array}$$

3. $\dfrac{40}{x} = \dfrac{20}{100}$

$$\dfrac{\overset{1}{\cancel{20}}x}{\underset{1}{\cancel{20}}} = \dfrac{4,000}{20}$$

$x = 200$

$$\begin{array}{r} 200 \\ 20\overline{)4,000} \\ -40 \\ \hline 000 \end{array}$$

4.

$$\dfrac{\dfrac{1}{2}}{\dfrac{3}{4}} = \dfrac{x}{100}$$

$$\dfrac{3}{4}x = \dfrac{1}{2} \cdot 100$$

$$\dfrac{\overset{1}{\cancel{4}}}{\underset{1}{\cancel{3}}} \cdot \dfrac{\overset{1}{\cancel{3}}}{\underset{1}{\cancel{4}}}x = \dfrac{50}{1} \cdot \dfrac{4}{3}$$

$$x = \dfrac{200}{3}$$

$$x = 66\dfrac{2}{3}\%$$

$$\begin{array}{r} 66\dfrac{2}{3} \\ 3\overline{)200} \\ -18 \\ \hline 20 \\ -18 \\ \hline 2 \end{array}$$

Section 4.3

5. $\dfrac{62.5}{100} \cdot \dfrac{10}{10} = \dfrac{\cancel{625}^{5}}{\cancel{1000}_{8}} = \dfrac{5}{8}$

6. $\dfrac{4}{5} = \dfrac{x}{100}$

$\dfrac{\cancel{5}^{1}x}{\cancel{5}_{1}} = \dfrac{400}{5}$

$x = 80\%$

$$5\overline{)400} \quad \begin{array}{r} 80 \\ \hline 400 \\ -40 \\ \hline 00 \end{array}$$

7. $\dfrac{8}{40} = \dfrac{x}{100}$

$\dfrac{\cancel{40}^{1}x}{\cancel{40}_{1}} = \dfrac{800}{40}$

$x = 20\%$

$$40\overline{)800} \quad \begin{array}{r} 20 \\ \hline 800 \\ -80 \\ \hline 00 \end{array}$$

Section 4.4

8. $500\% = 500. = 5$ 9. $7.98 = 7.98 = 798\%$

10. $\dfrac{8.6}{40\%} = \dfrac{8.6}{40.} = \dfrac{8.6}{0.40} = \dfrac{8.6}{0.4} = 21.5$

$$0.4\overline{)8.6.0} \quad \begin{array}{r} 21.5 \\ \hline 8.6.0 \\ -8 \\ \hline 06 \\ -4 \\ \hline 20 \\ -20 \\ \hline 0 \end{array}$$

4.1 Practice Ratios and Proportions

1. $\dfrac{2}{7} = \dfrac{x}{42}$

$\dfrac{\cancel{7}^{1}x}{\cancel{7}_{1}} = \dfrac{\cancel{84}^{12}}{\cancel{7}_{1}}$

$x = 12$

2. $\dfrac{3}{2} = \dfrac{12}{y}$

$\dfrac{\cancel{3}^{1}y}{\cancel{3}_{1}} = \dfrac{\cancel{24}^{8}}{\cancel{3}_{1}}$

$y = 8$

3. $\dfrac{k}{8} = \dfrac{8}{9}$

$\dfrac{\cancel{9}^{1}k}{\cancel{9}_{1}} = \dfrac{64}{9}$

$k = \dfrac{64}{9} = 7\dfrac{1}{9}$

4. $\dfrac{6}{z} = \dfrac{3}{5}$

$\dfrac{\cancel{3}^{1}z}{\cancel{3}_{1}} = \dfrac{\cancel{30}^{10}}{\cancel{3}_{1}}$

$z = 10$

5. $\dfrac{2}{5} = \dfrac{3}{w}$

$\dfrac{\cancel{2}^{1}w}{\cancel{2}_{1}} = \dfrac{15}{2}$

$w = \dfrac{15}{2} = 7\dfrac{1}{2}$

6. $\dfrac{x}{3} = \dfrac{3}{2}$

$\dfrac{\cancel{2}^{1}x}{\cancel{2}_{1}} = \dfrac{9}{2}$

$x = \dfrac{9}{2} = 4\dfrac{1}{2}$

7. $\dfrac{3}{5} = \dfrac{15}{n}$

$\dfrac{\cancel{3}^1 n}{\cancel{3}_1} = \dfrac{\cancel{75}^{25}}{\cancel{3}_1}$

$n = 25$

8. $\dfrac{1}{4} = \dfrac{x}{44}$

$\dfrac{\cancel{4}^1 x}{\cancel{4}_1} = \dfrac{\cancel{44}^{11}}{\cancel{4}_1}$

$x = 11$

9. $\dfrac{n}{5} = \dfrac{6}{15}$

$\dfrac{\cancel{15}^1 n}{\cancel{15}_1} = \dfrac{\cancel{30}^2}{\cancel{15}_1}$

$n = 2$

10. $\dfrac{3}{4} = \dfrac{16}{n}$

$\dfrac{\cancel{3}^1 n}{\cancel{3}_1} = \dfrac{64}{3}$

$n = \dfrac{64}{3} = 21\dfrac{1}{3}$

11. $\dfrac{n}{9} = \dfrac{1}{3}$

$\dfrac{\cancel{3}^1 n}{\cancel{3}_1} = \dfrac{\cancel{9}^3}{\cancel{3}_1}$

$n = 3$

12. $\dfrac{3}{x} = \dfrac{15}{25}$

$\dfrac{\cancel{15}^1 x}{\cancel{15}_1} = \dfrac{\cancel{75}^5}{\cancel{15}_1}$

$x = 5$

13. $\dfrac{3}{24} = \dfrac{k}{8}$

$\dfrac{\cancel{24}^1 k}{\cancel{24}_1} = \dfrac{\cancel{24}^1}{\cancel{24}_1}$

$k = 1$

14. $\dfrac{n}{32} = \dfrac{15}{16}$

$\dfrac{\cancel{16}^1 n}{\cancel{16}_1} = \dfrac{\cancel{480}^{30}}{\cancel{16}_1}$

$n = 30$

15. $\dfrac{7}{10} = \dfrac{20}{x}$

$\dfrac{\cancel{7}^1 x}{\cancel{7}_1} = \dfrac{200}{7}$

$x = \dfrac{200}{7} = 28\dfrac{4}{7}$

16. $\dfrac{x}{9} = \dfrac{25}{100}$

$\dfrac{\cancel{100}^1 x}{\cancel{100}_1} = \dfrac{\cancel{225}^9}{\cancel{100}_4}$

$x = \dfrac{9}{4} = 2\dfrac{1}{4}$

17. $\dfrac{9}{n} = \dfrac{3}{20}$

$\dfrac{\cancel{3}^1 n}{\cancel{3}_1} = \dfrac{\cancel{180}^{60}}{\cancel{3}_1}$

$n = 60$

18. $\dfrac{n}{10} = \dfrac{2}{5}$

$\dfrac{\cancel{5}^1 n}{\cancel{5}_1} = \dfrac{\cancel{20}^4}{\cancel{5}_1}$

$n = 4$

19. $\dfrac{16}{n} = \dfrac{7}{25}$

$\dfrac{\cancel{7}^1 n}{\cancel{7}_1} = \dfrac{400}{7}$

$n = \dfrac{400}{7} = 57\dfrac{1}{7}$

20. $\dfrac{3}{n} = \dfrac{7}{25}$

$\dfrac{\cancel{7}^1 n}{\cancel{7}_1} = \dfrac{75}{7}$

$n = \dfrac{75}{7}$

4.2 Practice the Percent Proportion

1. $\dfrac{x}{60} = \dfrac{30}{100}$

   $100x = 30 \cdot 60$

   $\dfrac{^1\cancel{100}x}{_1\cancel{100}} = \dfrac{\cancel{1,800}^{18}}{\cancel{100}_1}$

   $x = 18$

   $\begin{array}{r} 18 \\ 100\overline{)1,800} \\ \underline{-1\,00} \\ 800 \\ \underline{-800} \\ 0 \end{array}$

2. $\dfrac{7}{35} = \dfrac{x}{100}$

   $35x = 7 \cdot 100$

   $\dfrac{^1\cancel{35}x}{_1\cancel{35}} = \dfrac{\cancel{700}^{20}}{\cancel{35}_1}$

   $x = 20\%$

   $\begin{array}{r} 20 \\ 35\overline{)700} \\ \underline{-70} \\ 00 \end{array}$

3. $\dfrac{70}{x} = \dfrac{20}{100}$

   $20x = 70 \cdot 100$

   $\dfrac{^1\cancel{20}x}{_1\cancel{20}} = \dfrac{\cancel{7,000}^{\,700\;350}}{\cancel{20}_{\;2\;1}}$

   $x = 350$

   $\begin{array}{r} 350 \\ 20\overline{)7,000} \\ \underline{-6\,0} \\ 1\,00 \\ \underline{-1\,00} \\ 00 \end{array}$

4. $\dfrac{x}{47} = \dfrac{3.2}{100}$

   $100x = 47 \cdot 3.2$

   $\dfrac{^1\cancel{100}x}{_1\cancel{100}} = \dfrac{150.4}{100}$

   $x = 1.504$

   $\begin{array}{r} 1.504 \\ 100\overline{)150.400} \\ \underline{-100} \\ 50\ 4 \\ \underline{-50\ 0} \\ 400 \\ \underline{-400} \\ 0 \end{array}$

5. $\dfrac{x}{52} = \dfrac{150}{100}$

   $100x = 52 \cdot 150$

   $\dfrac{^1\cancel{100}x}{_1\cancel{100}} = \dfrac{\cancel{7,800}^{78}}{\cancel{100}_1}$

   $x = 78$

   $\begin{array}{r} 78 \\ 100\overline{)7,800} \\ \underline{-7\,00} \\ 800 \\ \underline{-800} \\ 0 \end{array}$

6. $\dfrac{x}{80} = \dfrac{0.4}{100}$

   $100x = 80 \cdot 0.4$

   $\dfrac{^1\cancel{100}x}{_1\cancel{100}} = \dfrac{32}{100}$

   $x = 0.32$

   $\begin{array}{r} 0.32 \\ 100\overline{)32.00} \\ \underline{-30\ 0} \\ 2\ 00 \\ \underline{-2\ 00} \\ 0 \end{array}$

7. *Work using fractions.*   **OR**   *Work using decimals.*

   $\dfrac{\frac{3}{5}}{2} = \dfrac{x}{100}$

   $2x = \dfrac{3}{_1\cancel{5}} \cdot \cancel{100}^{20}$

   $\dfrac{^1\cancel{2}x}{_1\cancel{2}} = \dfrac{\cancel{60}^{30}}{\cancel{2}_1}$

   $x = 30\%$

   Change $\dfrac{3}{5}$ to a decimal.

   $\begin{array}{r} 0.6 \\ 5\overline{)3.0} \\ \underline{-3\ 0} \\ 0 \end{array}$

   Work using decimals.

   $\dfrac{0.6}{2} = \dfrac{x}{100}$

   $2x = 0.6 \cdot 100$

   $\dfrac{^1\cancel{2}x}{_1\cancel{2}} = \dfrac{\cancel{60}^{30}}{\cancel{2}_1}$

   $x = 30\%$

8. $\dfrac{7}{x} = \dfrac{35}{100}$

$35x = 7 \cdot 100$

$\dfrac{{}^1\cancel{35}x}{{}_1\cancel{35}} = \dfrac{\cancel{100}\,{}^{20}}{\cancel{35}\,{}_1}$

$x = 20$

$\begin{array}{r} {}^120 \\ 35\overline{)700} \\ \underline{-70} \\ 00 \end{array}$

9. $\dfrac{135.08}{614} = \dfrac{x}{100}$

$614x = 100 \cdot 135.08$

$\dfrac{{}^1\cancel{614}x}{{}_1\cancel{614}} = \dfrac{13,508}{614}$

$x = 22\%$

$\begin{array}{r} 22 \\ 614\overline{)13,508} \\ \underline{-12\ 28} \\ 1\ 228 \\ \underline{-1\ 228} \\ 0 \end{array}$

10. $\dfrac{979.2}{x} = \dfrac{54.4}{100}$

$54.4x = 979.2 \cdot 100$

$\dfrac{{}^1\cancel{54.4}x}{{}_1\cancel{54.4}} = \dfrac{97,920}{54.4}$

$x = 1,800$

$\begin{array}{r} {}^{33}1{,}800. = 1{,}800 \\ 54.4\overline{)97{,}920.0.} \\ \underline{-54\ 4} \\ 43\ 52 \\ \underline{-43\ 52} \\ 00\ 0 \end{array}$

11. *Work using decimals.* $37\frac{1}{2} = 37\frac{5}{10} = 37.5$

$\dfrac{61.2}{x} = \dfrac{37.5}{100}$

$37.5x = 61.2 \cdot 100$

$\dfrac{{}^1\cancel{37.5}x}{{}_1\cancel{37.5}} = \dfrac{6,120}{37.5}$

$x = 163.2$

$\begin{array}{r} {}^{11}_{21}\\ {}^{43} 163.2 \\ 37.5\overline{)6{,}120.0.0} \\ \underline{-3\ 75} \\ 2\ 370 \\ \underline{-2\ 250} \\ 120\ 0 \\ \underline{-112\ 5} \\ 7\ 5\ 0 \\ \underline{-7\ 5\ 0} \\ 0 \end{array}$

OR

Work using fractions. $61.2 = 61\frac{2}{10} = 61\frac{1}{5}$

$\dfrac{61\frac{1}{5}}{x} = \dfrac{37\frac{1}{2}}{100}$

$37\frac{1}{2}x = 61\frac{1}{5} \cdot 100$

$\dfrac{{}^1\cancel{2}}{{}_1\cancel{75}} \cdot \dfrac{\cancel{75}^{\,1}}{\cancel{2}_1}x = \dfrac{306}{\cancel{5}_1} \cdot \dfrac{\cancel{100}^{\,20\ 4}}{1} \cdot \dfrac{2}{\cancel{75}_{15}}$

$x = \dfrac{2,448}{15} = 163\frac{1}{5}$

$\begin{array}{r} {}^1_3 163\frac{3}{15} = 163\frac{1}{5} \\ 15\overline{)2{,}448} \\ \underline{-15} \\ 94 \\ \underline{-90} \\ 48 \\ \underline{-45} \\ 3 \end{array}$

12. $\dfrac{16.2}{45} = \dfrac{x}{100}$

$45x = 16.2 \cdot 100$

$\dfrac{\cancel{45}x}{\cancel{45}} = \dfrac{1,620}{45}$

$x = 36\%$

$\begin{array}{r} 36 \\ 45\overline{)1,620} \\ \underline{-1\,35} \\ 270 \\ \underline{-270} \\ 0 \end{array}$

13. $\dfrac{x}{22.4} = \dfrac{35}{100}$

$100x = 35 \cdot 22.4$

$\dfrac{\cancel{100}x}{\cancel{100}} = \dfrac{784}{100}$

$x = 7.84$

$\begin{array}{r} 7.84 \\ 100\overline{)784.00} \\ \underline{-700} \\ 840 \\ \underline{-800} \\ 400 \\ \underline{-400} \\ 0 \end{array}$

14. $\dfrac{34.3}{49} = \dfrac{x}{100}$

$49x = 34.3 \cdot 100$

$\dfrac{\cancel{49}x}{\cancel{49}} = \dfrac{3,430}{49}$

$x = 70\%$

$\begin{array}{r} 70 \\ 49\overline{)3,430} \\ \underline{-3\,43} \\ 00 \end{array}$

15. $\dfrac{119.6}{x} = \dfrac{23}{100}$

$23x = 119.6 \cdot 100$

$\dfrac{\cancel{23}x}{\cancel{23}} = \dfrac{11,960}{23}$

$x = 520$

$\begin{array}{r} 520 \\ 23\overline{)11,960} \\ \underline{-11\,5} \\ 46 \\ \underline{-46} \\ 00 \end{array}$

16. $\dfrac{x}{700} = \dfrac{12}{100}$

$100x = 12 \cdot 700$

$\dfrac{\cancel{100}x}{\cancel{100}} = \dfrac{8,400}{100}$

$x = 84$

$\begin{array}{r} 84 \\ 100\overline{)8,400} \\ \underline{-8\,00} \\ 400 \\ \underline{-400} \\ 0 \end{array}$

17. $\dfrac{9.5}{x} = \dfrac{25}{100}$

$25x = 9.5 \cdot 100$

$\dfrac{\cancel{25}x}{\cancel{25}} = \dfrac{950}{25}$

$x = 38$

$\begin{array}{r} 38 \\ 25\overline{)950} \\ \underline{-75} \\ 200 \\ \underline{-200} \\ 0 \end{array}$

18. $\dfrac{3}{x} = \dfrac{\frac{5}{9}}{100}$

$\dfrac{5}{9}x = 3 \cdot 100$

$\dfrac{\cancel{9}}{\cancel{5}} \cdot \dfrac{\cancel{5}}{\cancel{9}}x = \dfrac{\cancel{300}^{60}}{1} \cdot \dfrac{9}{\cancel{5}}$

$x = 540$

19. $\dfrac{33}{x} = \dfrac{16.5}{100}$

$16.5x = 33 \cdot 100$

$\dfrac{\cancel{16.5}x}{\cancel{16.5}} = \dfrac{3,300}{16.5}$

$x = 200$

$\begin{array}{r} 20\,0 \\ 16.5\overline{)3,300.0.} \\ \underline{-3\,30} \\ 00\,0 \end{array}$

20. *Work using fractions.*

$\dfrac{66\frac{3}{5}}{360} = \dfrac{x}{100}$

$360x = 66\frac{3}{5} \cdot 100$

$\dfrac{1}{\cancel{360}} \cdot \dfrac{\cancel{360}^{1}}{1}x = \dfrac{333}{\cancel{5}} \cdot \dfrac{\cancel{100}^{20}}{1} \cdot \dfrac{1}{\cancel{360}_{18}}$

$x = \dfrac{333}{18} = 18\dfrac{9}{18} = 18\dfrac{1}{2}\%$

$\begin{array}{r} 18\frac{9}{18} = 18\frac{1}{2} \\ 18\overline{)333} \\ \underline{-18} \\ 153 \\ \underline{-144} \\ 9 \end{array}$

OR

Continued

Work using decimals.

Change $66\frac{3}{5}$ to a decimal number.

Write $\frac{3}{5}$ as a decimal. $5\overline{)3.0}$ $\;0.6$

50, $66\frac{3}{5} = 66.6$

$$\frac{66.6}{360} = \frac{x}{100}$$

$360x = 66.6 \cdot 100$

$$\frac{\cancel{360}^{1}x}{\cancel{360}_{1}} = \frac{6{,}660}{360}$$

$x = 18.5\%$

$\begin{array}{r} 18.5 \\ 360\overline{)6{,}660.0} \\ \underline{-3\,60} \\ 3\,060 \\ \underline{-2\,880} \\ 180\,0 \\ \underline{-180\,0} \\ 0 \end{array}$ ${}^{3}_{4}$

4.3 Practice Fractions, Ratios, and Percents

1. $50\% = \dfrac{\cancel{50}^{1}}{\cancel{100}_{2}} = \dfrac{1}{2}$

2. $74.25\% = \dfrac{74.25}{100} \cdot \dfrac{100}{100} = \dfrac{\cancel{7{,}425}^{297}}{\cancel{10{,}000}_{400}} = \dfrac{297}{400}$

3. $12.5\% = \dfrac{12.5}{100} \cdot \dfrac{10}{10} = \dfrac{\cancel{125}^{1}}{\cancel{1{,}000}_{8}} = \dfrac{1}{8}$

4. $60\% = \dfrac{\cancel{60}^{3}}{\cancel{100}_{5}} = \dfrac{3}{5}$

5. $165\% = \dfrac{\cancel{165}^{33}}{\cancel{100}_{20}} = \dfrac{33}{20} = 1\dfrac{13}{20}$

6. $45.375\% = \dfrac{45.375}{100} \cdot \dfrac{1{,}000}{1{,}000} = \dfrac{\cancel{45{,}375}^{363}}{\cancel{100{,}000}_{800}} = \dfrac{363}{800}$

7. $\dfrac{1}{2} = \dfrac{x}{100}$

$$\frac{\cancel{2}^{1}x}{\cancel{2}_{1}} = \frac{100}{2}$$

$x = 50\%$

$\begin{array}{r} 50 \\ 2\overline{)100} \\ \underline{-100} \\ 0 \end{array}$

8. $\dfrac{19}{10} = \dfrac{x}{100}$

$$\frac{\cancel{10}^{1}x}{\cancel{10}_{1}} = \frac{1{,}900}{10}$$

$x = 190\%$

$\begin{array}{r} 190 \\ 10\overline{)1{,}900} \\ \underline{-1\,0} \\ 90 \\ \underline{-90} \\ 00 \end{array}$

9. $\dfrac{2}{3} = \dfrac{x}{100}$

$\dfrac{\cancel{3}^{1}x}{\cancel{3}_{1}} = \dfrac{200}{3}$

$x = 66\dfrac{2}{3}\%$

$3\overline{)200}\;\;66\dfrac{2}{3}$
$\underline{-18}$
$\;\;20$
$\underline{-18}$
$\;\;\;2$

10. $\dfrac{1}{6} = \dfrac{x}{100}$

$\dfrac{\cancel{6}^{1}x}{\cancel{6}_{1}} = \dfrac{100}{6}$

$x = 16\dfrac{2}{3}\%$

$6\overline{)100}\;\;16\dfrac{4}{6} = 16\dfrac{2}{3}$
$\underline{-6}$
$\;\;40$
$\underline{-36}$
$\;\;\;4$

11. $\dfrac{11}{8} = \dfrac{x}{100}$

$\dfrac{\cancel{8}^{1}x}{\cancel{8}_{1}} = \dfrac{1{,}100}{8}$

$x = 137\dfrac{1}{2}\%$

$8\overline{)1{,}100}\;\;137\dfrac{4}{8} = 137\dfrac{1}{2}$
$\underline{-8}$
$\;\;30$
$\underline{-24}$
$\;\;60$
$\underline{-56}$
$\;\;\;4$

12. $\dfrac{3}{5} = \dfrac{x}{100}$

$\dfrac{\cancel{5}^{1}x}{\cancel{5}_{1}} = \dfrac{300}{5}$

$x = 60\%$

$5\overline{)300}\;\;60$
$\underline{-30}$
$\;\;00$

13. $\dfrac{7}{25} = \dfrac{x}{100}$

$\dfrac{\cancel{25}^{1}x}{\cancel{25}_{1}} = \dfrac{700}{25}$

$x = 28\%$

$25\overline{)700}\;\;\overset{4}{\underset{1}{}}28$
$\underline{-50}$
$\;\;200$
$\underline{-200}$
$\;\;\;\;0$

14. $\dfrac{7}{4} = \dfrac{x}{100}$

$\dfrac{\cancel{4}^{1}x}{\cancel{4}_{1}} = \dfrac{700}{4}$

$x = 175\%$

$4\overline{)700}\;\;175$
$\underline{-4}$
$\;\;30$
$\underline{-28}$
$\;\;20$
$\underline{-20}$
$\;\;\;0$

15. $3:8$ $\quad \dfrac{3}{8} = \dfrac{x}{100}$

$\dfrac{\cancel{8}^{1}x}{\cancel{8}_{1}} = \dfrac{300}{8}$

$x = 37\dfrac{1}{2}\%$

$8\overline{)300}\;\;37\dfrac{4}{8} = 37\dfrac{1}{2}$
$\underline{-24}$
$\;\;60$
$\underline{-56}$
$\;\;\;4$

16. $14:30$ $\quad \dfrac{14}{30} = \dfrac{x}{100}$

$\dfrac{\cancel{30}^{1}x}{\cancel{30}_{1}} = \dfrac{1{,}400}{30}$

$x = 46\dfrac{2}{3}\%$

$30\overline{)1{,}400}\;\;46\dfrac{20}{30} = 46\dfrac{2}{3}$
$\underline{-1\,20}$
$\;\;200$
$\underline{-180}$
$\;\;20$

17. $9:10$ $\dfrac{9}{10} = \dfrac{x}{100}$ $10\overline{)900}$
$\dfrac{\cancel{10}^{1}\,x}{\cancel{10}_{1}} = \dfrac{900}{10}$ $\dfrac{-90}{00}$

$x = 90\%$

18. $2:50$ $\dfrac{2}{50} = \dfrac{x}{100}$ $50\overline{)200}$
$\dfrac{\cancel{50}^{1}\,x}{\cancel{50}_{1}} = \dfrac{200}{50}$ $\dfrac{-200}{0}$

$x = 4\%$

19. $3:25$ $\dfrac{3}{25} = \dfrac{x}{100}$ $25\overline{)300}$
$\dfrac{\cancel{25}^{1}\,x}{\cancel{25}_{1}} = \dfrac{300}{25}$ $\dfrac{-25}{50}$ $\dfrac{-50}{0}$

$x = 12\%$

20. $12:20$ $\dfrac{12}{20} = \dfrac{x}{100}$ $20\overline{)1{,}200}$
$\dfrac{\cancel{20}^{1}\,x}{\cancel{20}_{1}} = \dfrac{1{,}200}{20}$ $\dfrac{-1\,20}{00}$

$x = 60\%$

4.4 Practice Decimals and Percents

1. $0.02 = 2\%$

2. $0.7 = 0.70 = 70\%$

3. $2.575 = 257.5\%$

4. $3 = 3.00 = 300\%$

5. $1.43 = 143\%$

6. $0.185 = 18.5\%$

7. $0.308 = 30.8\%$

8. $25\% = 25. = 0.25$

9. $1\% = 01. = 0.01$

10. $130\% = 130. = 1.30 = 1.3$

11. $52.5\% = 52.5 = 0.525$

12. $88\% = 88. = 0.88$

13. $425\% = 425. = 4.25$

14. $75.25\% = 75.25 = 0.7525$

15. $\dfrac{153}{45\%} = \dfrac{153}{45.} = \dfrac{153}{0.45} = 340$

$3\,40. = 340$

$0.45\overline{)153.00.}$
$\dfrac{-135}{18\,0}$
$\dfrac{-18\,0}{00}$

16. $\dfrac{4.4}{20\%} = \dfrac{4.4}{20.} = \dfrac{4.4}{0.20} = \dfrac{4.4}{0.2} = 22$

$2\,2. = 22$

$0.2\overline{)4.4.}$
$\dfrac{-4}{04}$
$\dfrac{-4}{0}$

17. $\dfrac{150}{40\%} = \dfrac{150}{40.} = \dfrac{150}{0.40} = \dfrac{150}{0.4} = 375$

18. $\dfrac{2.7}{45\%} = \dfrac{2.7}{45.} = \dfrac{2.7}{0.45} = 6$

$$\begin{array}{r} 2 \\ 2 \\ 1 \\ \end{array} \quad 375. = 375$$

$$0.4\overline{)150.0.}$$
$$\underline{-12}$$
$$30$$
$$\underline{-28}$$
$$20$$
$$\underline{-20}$$
$$0$$

$$6. = 6$$
$$0.45\overline{)2.70.}$$
$$\underline{-270}$$
$$0$$

19. $\dfrac{6.48}{36\%} = \dfrac{6.48}{36.} = \dfrac{6.48}{0.36} = 18$

20. $\dfrac{20}{100\%} = \dfrac{20}{100.} = \dfrac{20}{1.00} = \dfrac{20}{1} = 20$

$$18. = 18$$
$$0.36\overline{)6.48.}$$
$$\underline{-36}$$
$$288$$
$$\underline{-288}$$
$$0$$

4.6 Chapter Test for Percents, Ratios, and Proportions

Section 4.1

1. $\dfrac{2}{5} = \dfrac{x}{45}$

$$\dfrac{\overset{1}{\cancel{5}}x}{\underset{1}{\cancel{5}}} = \dfrac{\overset{18}{\cancel{90}}}{\underset{1}{\cancel{5}}}$$

$$x = 18$$

2. $\dfrac{x}{4} = \dfrac{36}{23}$

$$\dfrac{\overset{1}{\cancel{23}}x}{\underset{1}{\cancel{23}}} = \dfrac{144}{23}$$

$$x = \dfrac{144}{23} = 6\dfrac{6}{23}$$

Section 4.2

3. $\dfrac{x}{24} = \dfrac{25}{100}$

$$100\overline{)600}$$
$$\underline{-600}$$
$$0$$

$$\dfrac{\overset{1}{\cancel{100}}x}{\underset{1}{\cancel{100}}} = \dfrac{600}{100}$$

$$x = 6$$

4. $\dfrac{125}{37.5} = \dfrac{x}{100}$

$\dfrac{\cancel{37.5}^1 \, x}{\cancel{37.5}_1} = \dfrac{12{,}500}{37.5}$

$x = 333.\overline{3}\%$

$\begin{array}{r} 21 \\ 21 \\ 21 \\ 21 \end{array}$ 333.3... or 333.$\overline{3}$

$37.5\overline{)12{,}500.0.0}$
  $-11\ 25$
    $1\ 250$
   $-1\ 125$
     $125\ 0$
    $-112\ 5$
      $125\ 0$
     $-1\ 125$
       125

5. $\dfrac{139.6}{x} = \dfrac{20}{100}$

$\dfrac{\cancel{20}^1 \, x}{\cancel{20}_1} = \dfrac{13{,}960}{20}$

$x = 698$

$\begin{array}{r} 698 \\ 20\overline{)13{,}960} \\ -12\ 0 \\ \hline 1\ 96 \\ -1\ 80 \\ \hline 160 \\ -160 \\ \hline 0 \end{array}$

6.   *OR*

$\dfrac{5}{x} = \dfrac{\frac{4}{5}}{100}$

$\dfrac{4}{5}x = 500$

$\dfrac{\cancel{5}^1}{\cancel{4}_1} \bullet \dfrac{\cancel{4}^1}{\cancel{5}_1}x = \dfrac{500}{1} \bullet \dfrac{5}{4}$

$x = \dfrac{2{,}500}{4} = 625$

$\begin{array}{r} 625 \\ 4\overline{)2{,}500} \\ -2\ 4 \\ \hline 10 \\ -8 \\ \hline 20 \\ -20 \\ \hline 0 \end{array}$

$\dfrac{4}{5} = 0.8$ $\begin{array}{r} 0.8 \\ 5\overline{)4.0} \\ -4\ 0 \\ \hline 0 \end{array}$

$\dfrac{5}{x} = \dfrac{0.8}{100}$

$\dfrac{\cancel{0.8}^1 \, x}{\cancel{0.8}_1} = \dfrac{500}{0.8}$

$x = \dfrac{500}{0.8} = 625$

$\begin{array}{r} 62\ 5.\ = 625 \\ 0.8\overline{)500.0.} \\ -48 \\ \hline 20 \\ -16 \\ \hline 4\ 0 \\ -4\ 0 \\ \hline 0 \end{array}$

7. *Work using fractions.*   *Work using decimals.*

$$\frac{\frac{1}{2}}{\frac{5}{4}} = \frac{x}{100}$$ OR $\frac{1}{2} = 0.5$ $2\overline{)1.0}$ $\frac{5}{4} = 1.25$ $4\overline{)5.00}$

$$\frac{0.5}{2\overline{)1.0}}$$ $$\frac{-1\ 0}{0}$$

$$\frac{1.25}{4\overline{)5.00}}$$ $$\frac{-4}{1\ 0}$$ $$\frac{-8}{20}$$ $$\frac{-20}{0}$$

$$\frac{5}{4}x = \frac{1}{2} \cdot \frac{100}{1}$$ ($\frac{100^{50}}{1 \cancel{2}}$)

$$\frac{\cancel{4}}{\cancel{5}} \cdot \frac{\cancel{5}}{\cancel{4}}x = \frac{50}{1} \cdot \frac{4}{5}$$

$$x = \frac{40}{1} = 40\%$$

$$\frac{0.5}{1.25} = \frac{x}{100}$$

$$1.25x = 0.5 \cdot 100$$

$$\frac{1.25x}{1.25} = \frac{50}{1.25}$$

$$x = 40\%$$

$$1.25\overline{)50.00.} \quad 40. = 40$$

$$\frac{-50\ 0}{00}$$

8. $$\frac{x}{600} = \frac{12.5}{100}$$ $$100\overline{)7,500}$$

$$\frac{75}{100\overline{)7,500}}$$ $$\frac{-7\ 00}{500}$$ $$\frac{-500}{0}$$

$$\frac{100\ x}{100} = \frac{7,500}{100}$$

$$x = 75$$

Section 4.3

9. $15\% = \frac{\cancel{15}^3}{\cancel{100}_{20}} = \frac{3}{20}$

10. $62.5\% = \frac{62.5}{100} \cdot \frac{10}{10} = \frac{\cancel{625}^5}{\cancel{1000}_8} = \frac{5}{8}$

11. $$\frac{9}{5} = \frac{x}{100}$$

$$\frac{\cancel{5}x}{\cancel{5}} = \frac{900}{5}$$

$$x = 180\%$$

$$\frac{180}{5\overline{)900}}$$ $$\frac{-5}{40}$$ $$\frac{-40}{00}$$

12. $$\frac{1}{3} = \frac{x}{100}$$

$$\frac{\cancel{3}x}{\cancel{3}} = \frac{100}{3}$$

$$x = 33\frac{1}{3}\%$$

$$\frac{33\frac{1}{3}}{3\overline{)100}}$$ $$\frac{-9}{10}$$ $$\frac{-9}{1}$$

13. $7 : 20$ $$\frac{7}{20} = \frac{x}{100}$$

$$\frac{\cancel{20}\ x}{\cancel{20}} = \frac{700}{20}$$

$$x = 35\%$$

$$\frac{35}{20\overline{)700}}$$ $$\frac{-60}{100}$$ $$\frac{-100}{0}$$

Section 4.4

14. $100\% = \underset{\smile\smile}{100.} = 1.\cancel{00} = 1$

15. $37.5\% = \underset{\smile\smile}{37.5} = 0.375$

16. $3.49 = \underset{\smile\smile}{3.49} = 349\%$

17. $7 = \underset{\smile\smile}{7.00} = 700\%$

18. $\dfrac{32}{20\%} = \dfrac{32}{\underset{\smile\smile}{20.}} = \dfrac{32}{0.2\cancel{0}} = \dfrac{32}{0.2} = 160$

$$
\begin{array}{r}
160. = 160 \\
0.2.\overline{\smash{)}32.0.} \\
\underline{-2} \\
12 \\
\underline{-12} \\
0\ 0
\end{array}
$$

19. $\dfrac{150}{10\%} = \dfrac{150}{\underset{\smile\smile}{10.}} = \dfrac{150}{0.1\cancel{0}} = \dfrac{150}{0.1} = 1{,}500$

$$
\begin{array}{r}
150\ 0. = 1{,}500 \\
0.1\overline{\smash{)}150.0.} \\
\underline{-1} \\
05 \\
\underline{-5} \\
0\ 0\ 0
\end{array}
$$

20. $\dfrac{50}{100\%} = \dfrac{50}{\underset{\smile\smile}{100.}} = \dfrac{50}{1.\cancel{00}} = \dfrac{50}{1} = 50$

5.0   Pretest for Positive and Negative Numbers

Section 5.1

1. $(-14) + (-9)$
   -23

   Negative + negative = negative.

2. $28 + (-13)$
   15

   a. Subtract 28 - 13 = 15.
   b. Larger number 28 is positive.
   c. The answer is +15.

Section 5.2

3. $17 - (-8)$
   17 + 8
   25

4. $3 - 27$
   3 + (-27)
   -24

Section 5.3

5. $3(-8)$ = -24   6. $\dfrac{-56}{-8}$ = 7

Section 5.4

7. $\underline{x^2 + 3x} \;\boxed{-1}\; \underline{-3x^2} \;\boxed{+4}$
   $-2x^2 + 3x + 3$

8. $\underline{3x^4} + \underline{2x^4} \;\boxed{-7}\;\boxed{-25}$
   $5x^4 - 32$

Section 5.5

9. $3(-2y - 7)$
   $-6y - 21$

10. $-(-x^2 + 5x - 9)$
   $-1(-x^2 + 5x - 9)$
   $x^2 - 5x + 9$

5.1 Practice Adding Positive and Negative Numbers

1. (−5) + 30

    25

a. Subtract 30 − 5 = 25.
b. Larger number 30 is positive.
c. The answer is +25.

2. (−8) + 6

    −2

a. Subtract 8 − 6 = 2.
b. Larger number 8 is negative.
c. The answer is −2.

3. (−9) + (−15)

    −24

Negative + negative = negative.

4. 30 + 5

    35

Positive + positive = positive.

5. (−8) + (−8)

    −16

Negative + negative = negative.

6. 40 + (−20)

    20

a. Subtract 40 − 20 = 20.
b. Larger number 40 is positive.
c. The answer is +20.

7. (−9) + 5

    −4

a. Subtract 9 − 5 = 4.
b. Larger number 9 is negative.
c. The answer is −4.

8. 7 + (−10)

    −3

a. Subtract 10 − 7 = 3.
b. Larger number 10 is negative.
c. The answer is −3.

9. 25 + 15

    40

Positive + positive = positive

10. 8 + (−9)

    −1

a. Subtract 9 − 8 = 1.
b. Larger number 9 is negative.
c. The answer is −1.

11. (−42) + (−36)

    −78

Negative + negative = negative.

12. 15 + 30

    45

Positive + positive = positive.

13. 4 + (−4)
  0

Any number + its opposite = 0.

14. 10 + (−20)
  −10

a. Subtract 20 − 10 = 10.
b. Larger number 20 is negative.
c. The answer is −10.

15. 4 + (−2)
  2

a. Subtract 4 − 2 = 2.
b. Larger number 4 is positive.
c. The answer is 2.

16. 6 + (−7)
  −1

a. Subtract 7 − 6 = 1.
b. Larger number 7 is negative.
c. The answer is −1.

17. (−5) + 9
  4

a. Subtract 9 − 5 = 4.
b. Larger number 9 is positive.
c. The answer is 4.

18. (−1) + (−1)
  −2

Negative + negative = negative.

19. (−14) + (−7)
  −21

Negative + negative = negative.

20. (−1,234) + 1,234
  0

Any number + its opposite = 0.

5.2 Practice Subtracting Positive and Negative Numbers

1. 31 − 12
 31 + (−12)
  19

2. 8 − 79
 8 + (−79)
  −71

3. 11 − 46
 11 + (−46)
  −35

4. (−15) − 65
 (−15) + (−65)
  −80

5. 14 − (−8)
 14 + 8
  22

6. (−19) − 17
 (−19) + (−17)
  −36

7. (−7) − (−31)
 (−7) + 31
  24

8. 12 − (−63)
 12 + 63
  75

9. (−61) − (−5)
 (−61) + 5
  −56

10. 69 − 18
 69 + (−18)
  51

11. (−9) − 7
 (−9) + (−7)
  −16

12. (−47) − (−28)
 (−47) + 28
  −19

13. 47 − 58
47 + (−58)
−11

14. (−9) − (−10)
(−9) + 10
1

15. (−19) − 5
(−19) + (−5)
−24

16. (−16) − (−18)
(−16) + 18
2

17. 31 − 17
31 + (−17)
14

18. (−11) − 6
(−11) + (−6)
−17

19. 99 − (−1)
99 + 1
100

20. (−8) − (−12)
(−8) + 12
4

5.3 Practice Multiplying and Dividing Positive and Negative Numbers

1. (−9)(1) = −9

2. 5(−1) = −5

3. (−10)(−4) = 40

4. (−7)(−4) = 28

5. (−5)(−2) = 10

6. (−2)(−4) = 8

7. 6(−8) = −48

8. 5(−4) = −20

9. (−14)(0) = 0

10. 8(4) = 32

11. $\dfrac{-77}{7}$ = −11

12. $\dfrac{81}{9}$ = 9

13. $\dfrac{-24}{-2}$ = 12

14. $\dfrac{48}{-6}$ = −8

15. $\dfrac{72}{-8}$ = −9

16. $\dfrac{-14}{-2}$ = 7

17. $\dfrac{-36}{6}$ = −6

18. $\dfrac{45}{-9}$ = −5

19. $\dfrac{35}{-5}$ = −7

20. $\dfrac{56}{8}$ = 7

5.4 Practice Collecting Like Terms

1. 4y − 8y
4y + (−8y)
−4y

2. (−9x) − 4x
(−9x) + (−4x)
−13x

3. −5b + 4b
−1b
−b

4. $5bx^2 - 2bx^2$
$5bx^2 + (-2bx^2)$
$3bx^2$

5. x − 8x
1x + (−8x)
−7x

6. (−6x) + 6x
0

7. $\underline{5a} + 2a^2 \underline{+ 6a}$
   $11a + 2a^2$

8. $\underline{4y + 3y} - 2xy$
   $7y - 2xy$

9. $\underline{3a^2 + 4a^2} + 5$
   $7a^2 + 5$

10. $-45a + 44a$
    $-1a$
    $-a$

11. $\underline{2x}\,\boxed{-3}\underline{+ 3x}\,\boxed{-2}$
    $5x - 5$

12. $\underline{6a^2 + 7a^2} + 8$
    $13a^2 + 8$

13. $\underline{3a} - 1 \underline{+ a} + 3b$
    $4a - 1 + 3b$

14. $\underline{-a} + 2 + 8a^2 - 7$
    $-a - 5 + 8a^2$

15. $\underline{-4x^2}\,\boxed{+ 8} - 5xy \underline{+ 2x^2}\,\boxed{- 10}$
    $-2x^2 - 2 - 5xy$

16. $\underline{-9x}\,\boxed{- x^2}\underline{+ x}\,\boxed{- 2x^2}+ 4$
    $-8x - 3x^2 + 4$

17. $-18a^2 + 17a^2$
    $-1a^2$
    $-a^2$

18. $\underline{(-5x)} + 6 \underline{- 3x}$
    $-8x + 6$

19. $\underline{7a^3}\,\boxed{+ 3}\underline{- 7a^3}\,\boxed{- 3}$
    0

20. $\underline{-6x^2} - 1 \underline{- x} - 10$
    $-6x^2 - 11 - x$

5.5 Practice the Distributive Property

1. $5(2x + 1)$
   $10x + 5$

2. $2(-4x - 3)$
   $-8x - 6$

3. $-7(-3y + 2)$
   $21y - 14$

4. $-3(5x^2 + 4x - 7)$
   $-15x^2 - 12x + 21$

5. $-3(2x^2 + x - 4)$
   $-6x^2 - 3x + 12$

6. $-4(-3x + 2)$
   $12x - 8$

7. $-(a + 1)$
   $-1(a + 1)$
   $-a - 1$

8. $-8(2a + 3)$
   $-16a - 24$

9. $-4(-x - 5)$
   $4x + 20$

10. $-7(4x^2 - 5x - 2)$
    $-28x^2 + 35x + 14$

11. $-9(2 - y)$
    $-18 + 9y$

12. $-(2x + 5)$
    $-1(2x + 5)$
    $-2x - 5$

13. $2(-x^3 + x^2 - 1)$
    $-2x^3 + 2x^2 - 2$

14. $-3(x - 2)$
    $-3x + 6$

15. $-(y - 2)$
    $-1(y - 2)$
    $-y + 2$

16. $-(-y + 5)$

$-1(-y + 5)$

$y - 5$

17. $3(x + y + 5)$

$3x + 3y + 15$

18. $-4(5y + 6x - 2)$

$-20y - 24x + 8$

19. $-2(x^2 + 3x - 4)$

$-2x^2 - 6x + 8$

20. $-(3x + 7y + 9)$

$-1(3x + 7y + 9)$

$-3x - 7y - 9$

5.6 Chapter Test for Positive and Negative Numbers

Section 5.1

1. $-6 + 12$

6

a. Subtract 12 - 6 = 6.
b. Larger number 12 is positive.
c. The answer is +6.

2. $-18 + 18$

0

Any number + its opposite = 0.

3. $6 + (-4)$

2

a. Subtract 6 - 4 = 2.
b. Larger number 6 is positive.
c. The answer is +2.

4. $-5 + (-29)$

-34

Negative + negative = negative.

Section 5.2

5. $32 - 13$

$32 + (-13)$

19

6. $(-8) - (-6)$

$(-8) + 6$

-2

7. $9 - 81$

$9 + (-81)$

-72

8. $(-14) - 67$

$(-14) + (-67)$

-81

Section 5.3

9. $7(-7)$ = -49

10. $(-9)(-11)$ = 99

11. $\dfrac{-27}{-3}$ = 9

12. $\dfrac{\cancel{14}^{2^{1}}}{\cancel{-42}_{6_{3}}}$ = $-\dfrac{1}{3}$

Section 5.4

13. $\underline{5a + 6a} - 7$
   $11a - 7$

14. $7xy + 4x - 8xy$
   $-xy + 4x$

15. $-10x \;(- 4) + 6x \;(- 10)$
   $-4x - 14$

16. $-5x^2 + 7x + 5x^2$
   $7x$

Section 5.5

17. $6(2x + 7y)$
   $12x + 42y$

18. $-4(3x - 6)$
   $-12x + 24$

19. $-2(x^2 + 6x - 4)$
   $-2x^2 - 12x + 8$

20. $-(-x^2 + 3x - 7)$
   $-1(-x^2 + 3x - 7)$
   $x^2 - 3x + 7$

SOLUTIONS

6.0 **Pretest for Equations**

Section 6.1

1. $x - 21 = -22$

   $\underline{+21 = +21}$

   $x = -1$

2. $-18 = x + 37$

   $x + 37 = -18$

   $\underline{-37 = -37}$

   $x = -55$

Section 6.2

3. $-12x = -60$

   $\dfrac{\overset{1}{-12}x}{\underset{1}{-12}} = \dfrac{\overset{5}{-60}}{\underset{1}{-12}}$

   $x = 5$

4. $\dfrac{-5x}{11} = 35$

   $\left(\dfrac{\overset{1}{-11}}{5}\right)\left(\dfrac{-5}{\underset{1}{11}}\right)^{1} x = \dfrac{\overset{7}{35}}{1} \cdot \left(\dfrac{-11}{5}\right)_{1}$

   $x = -77$

Section 6.3

5. $-64 = 6x + 14$

   $6x + 14 = -64$

   $\underline{-14 = -14}$

   $\dfrac{\overset{1}{6}x}{\underset{1}{6}} = \dfrac{\overset{13}{-78}}{6}_{1}$

   $x = -13$

6. $53 - \dfrac{5}{8}x = -102$

   $\underline{-53 \qquad\qquad = -53}$

   $-\dfrac{5}{8}x = -155$

   $\left(-\dfrac{\overset{1}{8}}{5}\right)\left(-\dfrac{5}{\underset{1}{8}}\right)^{1} x = \left(\dfrac{\overset{31}{-155}}{1}\right)\left(-\dfrac{8}{5}\right)$

   $x = 248$

Section 6.4

7. $-12n + 84 = -8n$

   $\underline{+8n \qquad\quad = +8n}$

   $-4n + 84 = 0$

   $\underline{-84 = -84}$

   $\dfrac{\overset{1}{-4}n}{\underset{1}{-4}} = \dfrac{\overset{21}{-84}}{-4}_{1}$

   $n = 21$

8. $3(x - 6) = 2(x + 3)$

   $3x - 18 = 2x + 6$

   $\underline{-2x \qquad\quad = -2x}$

   $x - 18 = 6$

   $\underline{+18 = +18}$

   $x = 24$

9. $4x - 4 + 5x - 3 = -4x - 46$

$$9x - 7 = \cancel{-4x} - 46$$
$$+4x = +4x$$
$$13x \cancel{-7} = -46$$
$$+7 = +7$$
$$\frac{^1\cancel{13}x}{_1\cancel{13}} = \frac{-39^3}{\cancel{13}_1}$$
$$x = -3$$

10. $4(a - 3) = 3 - (a + 5)$

$$4a - 12 = 3 - a - 5$$
$$4a - 12 = \cancel{-a} - 2$$
$$+a = +a$$
$$5a \cancel{-12} = -2$$
$$\cancel{+12} = +12$$
$$\frac{^1\cancel{5}a}{_1\cancel{5}} = \frac{\cancel{10}^2}{\cancel{5}_1}$$
$$a = 2$$

6.1 Practice Solving Equations by Adding and Subtracting

1. $x + 9 = 10$
$$\cancel{-9} = -9$$
$$x = 1$$

2. $x - 3 = -8$
$$+3 = +3$$
$$x = -5$$

3. $y - 6 = 4$
$$+6 = +6$$
$$y = 10$$

4. $x + 5 = -10$
$$\cancel{-5} = -5$$
$$x = -15$$

5. $4 = b + 7$
$$b + 7 = 4$$
$$\cancel{-7} = -7$$
$$b = -3$$

6. $y + 11 = -6$
$$\cancel{-11} = -11$$
$$y = -17$$

7. $x - 7 = -5$
$$+7 = +7$$
$$x = 2$$

8. $s - 4 = 10$
$$+4 = +4$$
$$s = 14$$

9. $-7 = x + 5$
$$x + 5 = -7$$
$$\cancel{-5} = -5$$
$$x = -12$$

10. $y + 15 = 10$
$$\cancel{-15} = -15$$
$$y = -5$$

11. $x + 4.1 = 9.2$
$$\cancel{-4.1} = -4.1$$
$$x = 5.1$$

12. $a - 3 = 12$
$$+3 = +3$$
$$a = 15$$

13. $x - 16 = 0$
$$\cancel{+16} = +16$$
$$x = 16$$

14. $x + 7.5 = -3.4$
$$\cancel{-7.5} = -7.5$$
$$x = -10.9$$

15. $x - 12 = -15$
$$\cancel{+12} = +12$$
$$x = -3$$

16. $51 = h - 22$
$$h - 22 = 51$$
$$\cancel{+22} = +22$$
$$h = 73$$

17. $x - 3 = -1$
$$+3 = +3$$
$$x = 2$$

18. $x + 5 = -14$
$$\cancel{-5} = -5$$
$$x = -19$$

19. $-3 = k - 8$

$$k - 8 = -3$$
$$\underline{+ 8 = +8}$$
$$k = 5$$

20. $x - 5 = 13$

$$\underline{+ 5 = +5}$$
$$x = 18$$

6.2 Practice Solving Equations by Multiplying and Dividing

1. $5x = 90$

$$\frac{\cancel{5}^{1}x}{\cancel{5}_{1}} = \frac{\cancel{90}^{18}}{\cancel{5}_{1}}$$
$$x = 18$$

2. $\dfrac{-m}{5} = 12$

$$\cancel{5}^{1} \cdot \frac{-m}{\cancel{5}_{1}} = 12 \cdot 5$$

$$\frac{-m}{-1} = \frac{60}{-1}$$

$$m = -60$$

3. $\dfrac{x}{10} = 25$

$$\cancel{10}^{1} \cdot \frac{x}{\cancel{10}_{1}} = 25 \cdot 10$$
$$x = 250$$

4. $86 = 2v$

$$2v = 86$$
$$\frac{\cancel{2}^{1}v}{\cancel{2}_{1}} = \frac{\cancel{86}^{43}}{\cancel{2}_{1}}$$
$$v = 43$$

5. $\dfrac{k}{-2} = 37$

$$\cancel{-2}^{1} \cdot \frac{k}{\cancel{-2}_{1}} = 37 \cdot (-2)$$

$$k = -74$$

6. $-12p = -132$

$$\frac{\cancel{-12}p}{\cancel{-12}} = \frac{\cancel{-132}^{11}}{\cancel{-12}_{1}}$$
$$p = 11$$

7. $\dfrac{-h}{7} = 20$

$$\cancel{7}^{1} \cdot \frac{-h}{\cancel{7}_{1}} = 20 \cdot 7$$

$$\frac{-h}{-1} = \frac{140}{-1}$$

$$h = -140$$

8. $95 = -5y$

$$-5y = 95$$
$$\frac{\cancel{-5}^{1}y}{\cancel{-5}_{1}} = \frac{\cancel{95}^{19}}{\cancel{-5}_{1}}$$
$$y = -19$$

9. $3m = -384$

$$\frac{\cancel{3}^{1}m}{\cancel{3}_{1}} = \frac{\cancel{-384}^{128}}{\cancel{3}_{1}}$$
$$m = -128$$

10. $-21r = 672$

$$\frac{\cancel{-21}^{1}r}{\cancel{-21}_{1}} = \frac{\cancel{672}^{32}}{\cancel{-21}_{1}}$$
$$r = -32$$

11. $\dfrac{x}{100} = 7$

$\overset{1}{\cancel{100}} \cdot \dfrac{x}{\cancel{100}_1} = 7 \cdot 100$

$x = 700$

12. $-3 = \dfrac{a}{45}$

$\dfrac{a}{45} = -3$

$\overset{1}{\cancel{45}} \cdot \dfrac{a}{\cancel{45}_1} = -3 \cdot 45$

$a = -135$

13. $-18p = -306$

$\dfrac{\overset{1}{\cancel{-18}}p}{{}_1\cancel{-18}} = \dfrac{\cancel{-306}^{17}}{\cancel{-18}_1}$

$p = 17$

14. $\dfrac{b}{-9} = -7$

$\overset{1}{\cancel{-9}} \cdot \dfrac{b}{\cancel{-9}_1} = -7 \cdot (-9)$

$b = 63$

15. $5x = -200$

$\dfrac{\overset{1}{\cancel{5}}x}{{}_1\cancel{5}} = \dfrac{\cancel{-200}^{40}}{\cancel{5}_1}$

$x = -40$

16. $-84 = \dfrac{2x}{7}$

$\dfrac{2x}{7} = -84$

$\dfrac{\overset{1}{\cancel{7}}}{{}_1\cancel{2}} \cdot \dfrac{\overset{1}{\cancel{2}}x}{\cancel{7}_1} = -\dfrac{\cancel{84}^{42}}{1} \cdot \dfrac{7}{\cancel{2}_1}$

$x = -294$

17. $\dfrac{-x}{4} = -4$

$\overset{1}{\cancel{4}} \cdot \dfrac{-x}{\cancel{4}_1} = -4 \cdot 4$

$\dfrac{-x}{-1} = \dfrac{-16}{-1}$

$x = 16$

18. $-4x = 120$

$\dfrac{\overset{1}{\cancel{-4}}x}{{}_1\cancel{-4}} = \dfrac{\cancel{120}^{30}}{\cancel{-4}_1}$

$x = -30$

19. $\dfrac{-3x}{8} = 24$

$\dfrac{-3}{8}x = 24$

$\overset{1}{\cancel{\left(\dfrac{-8}{3}\right)}}{}_1 \overset{1}{\cancel{\left(\dfrac{-3}{8}\right)}}{}_1 x = \dfrac{\overset{8}{\cancel{24}}}{1}\left(\dfrac{-8}{\cancel{3}}\right)_1$

$x = -64$

20. $-12y = -156$

$\dfrac{\overset{1}{\cancel{-12}}y}{{}_1\cancel{-12}} = \dfrac{\cancel{-156}^{13}}{\cancel{-12}_1}$

$y = 13$

6.3 Practice Solving Two-Step Equations

1. $4d + 5 = 85$

$\quad\quad -5 = -5$

$\quad\quad \dfrac{4d}{4} = \dfrac{80}{4}$

$\quad\quad\quad d = 20$

2. $2r - 7 = 1$

$\quad\quad +7 = +7$

$\quad\quad \dfrac{2r}{2} = \dfrac{8}{2}$

$\quad\quad\quad r = 4$

3. $-8 = -2b + 4$

$\quad\quad -2b + 4 = -8$

$\quad\quad\quad\quad -4 = -4$

$\quad\quad \dfrac{-2b}{-2} = \dfrac{-12}{-2}$

$\quad\quad\quad b = 6$

4. $\dfrac{1}{6}x + 9 = 12$

$\quad\quad -9 = -9$

$\quad\quad \dfrac{1}{6}x = 3$

$\quad\quad \dfrac{6}{1} \cdot \dfrac{1}{6}x = 3 \cdot \dfrac{6}{1}$

$\quad\quad\quad x = 18$

5. $\dfrac{b}{7} + 7 = 19$

$\quad\quad -7 = -7$

$\quad\quad \dfrac{b}{7} = 12$

$\quad\quad \dfrac{7}{1} \cdot \dfrac{b}{7} = 12 \cdot 7$

$\quad\quad\quad b = 84$

6. $\dfrac{x}{4} - 12 = 9$

$\quad\quad +12 = +12$

$\quad\quad \dfrac{x}{4} = 21$

$\quad\quad \dfrac{4}{1} \cdot \dfrac{x}{4} = 21 \cdot 4$

$\quad\quad\quad x = 84$

7. $-t - 8 = -25$

$\quad\quad +8 = +8$

$\quad\quad -t = -17$

$\quad\quad \dfrac{-t}{-1} = \dfrac{-17}{-1}$

$\quad\quad\quad t = 17$

8. $-7m + 1.2 = 4.0$

$\quad\quad -1.2 = -1.2$

$\quad\quad -7m = 2.8$

$\quad\quad \dfrac{-7m}{-7} = \dfrac{2.8}{-7}$

$\quad\quad\quad m = -0.4$

9. $9 = \dfrac{n}{4} - 3$

$\quad\quad \dfrac{n}{4} - 3 = 9$

$\quad\quad\quad\quad +3 = +3$

$\quad\quad \dfrac{n}{4} = 12$

$\quad\quad \dfrac{4}{1} \cdot \dfrac{n}{4} = 12 \cdot 4$

$\quad\quad\quad n = 48$

10. $\dfrac{y}{3} + 6 = -45$

$\quad\quad -6 = -6$

$\quad\quad \dfrac{y}{3} = -51$

$\quad\quad \dfrac{3}{1} \cdot \dfrac{y}{3} = -51 \cdot 3$

$\quad\quad\quad y = -153$

11. $\dfrac{-p}{3} + 13 = -4$

$\quad\quad -13 = -13$

$\quad\quad \dfrac{-p}{3} = -17$

$\quad\quad \dfrac{3}{1} \cdot \dfrac{-p}{3} = -17 \cdot 3$

$\quad\quad \dfrac{-p}{-1} = \dfrac{-51}{-1}$

$\quad\quad\quad p = 51$

12. $-y + 0.6 = 1.8$

$\quad\quad -0.6 = -0.6$

$\quad\quad -y = 1.2$

$\quad\quad \dfrac{-y}{-1} = \dfrac{1.2}{-1}$

$\quad\quad\quad y = -1.2$

13. $\dfrac{2x}{5} + \cancel{17} = 9$

$$\underline{\quad \cancel{17} = -17 \quad}$$

$$\dfrac{2x}{5} = -8$$

$$\dfrac{\overset{1}{\cancel{5}}}{\underset{1}{\cancel{2}}} \cdot \dfrac{\overset{1}{\cancel{2}}}{\underset{1}{\cancel{5}}}x = \dfrac{\overset{4}{\cancel{-8}}}{1} \cdot \dfrac{5}{\underset{1}{\cancel{2}}}$$

$$x = -20$$

14. $2 = 14 - \dfrac{3}{4}x$

$$\cancel{14} - \dfrac{3}{4}x = 2$$

$$\underline{\quad -\cancel{14} \qquad = -14 \quad}$$

$$-\dfrac{3}{4}x = -12$$

$$\left(-\dfrac{\overset{1}{\cancel{4}}}{\underset{1}{\cancel{3}}}\right)\left(-\dfrac{\overset{1}{\cancel{3}}}{\underset{1}{\cancel{4}}}\right)x = -\dfrac{\overset{4}{\cancel{12}}}{1}\left(-\dfrac{4}{\cancel{3}}\right)_1$$

$$x = 16$$

15. $-5x - \cancel{12} = -2$

$$\underline{\quad \cancel{12} = +12 \quad}$$

$$-5x = 10$$

$$\dfrac{\overset{1}{\cancel{-5}}x}{\underset{1}{\cancel{-5}}} = \dfrac{\overset{2}{\cancel{10}}}{\underset{1}{\cancel{-5}}}$$

$$x = -2$$

16. $-2x + \cancel{3} = 2$

$$\underline{\quad -\cancel{3} = -3 \quad}$$

$$-2x = -1$$

$$\dfrac{\overset{1}{\cancel{-2}}x}{\underset{1}{\cancel{-2}}} = \dfrac{-1}{-2}$$

$$x = \dfrac{1}{2}$$

17. $\cancel{67} - \dfrac{3}{4}x = 85$

$$\underline{\quad -\cancel{67} \qquad = -67 \quad}$$

$$-\dfrac{3}{4}x = 18$$

$$\left(-\dfrac{\overset{1}{\cancel{4}}}{\underset{1}{\cancel{3}}}\right)\left(-\dfrac{\overset{1}{\cancel{3}}}{\underset{1}{\cancel{4}}}\right)x = \dfrac{\overset{6}{\cancel{18}}}{1}\left(-\dfrac{4}{\cancel{3}}\right)_1$$

$$x = -24$$

18. $\dfrac{2}{3}x - \cancel{9} = 11$

$$\underline{\quad +\cancel{9} = +9 \quad}$$

$$\dfrac{2}{3}x = 20$$

$$\dfrac{\overset{1}{\cancel{3}}}{\underset{1}{\cancel{2}}} \cdot \dfrac{\overset{1}{\cancel{2}}}{\underset{1}{\cancel{3}}}x = \dfrac{\overset{10}{\cancel{20}}}{1} \cdot \dfrac{3}{\underset{1}{\cancel{2}}}$$

$$x = 30$$

19. $2 = -3x - 10$

$$-3x - \cancel{10} = 2$$

$$\underline{\quad +\cancel{10} = +10 \quad}$$

$$-3x = 12$$

$$\dfrac{\overset{1}{\cancel{-3}}x}{\underset{1}{\cancel{-3}}} = \dfrac{\overset{4}{\cancel{12}}}{\underset{1}{\cancel{-3}}}$$

$$x = -4$$

20. $\dfrac{5}{7}x - \cancel{13} = 82$

$$\underline{\quad +\cancel{13} = +13 \quad}$$

$$\dfrac{5}{7}x = 95$$

$$\dfrac{\overset{1}{\cancel{7}}}{\underset{1}{\cancel{5}}} \cdot \dfrac{\overset{1}{\cancel{5}}}{\underset{1}{\cancel{7}}}x = \dfrac{\overset{19}{\cancel{95}}}{1} \cdot \dfrac{7}{\underset{1}{\cancel{5}}}$$

$$x = 133$$

6.4 Practice Solving Equations When a Variable Occurs Multiple Times

1. $-9x - 72 = 3x$

$\underline{-3x \qquad = -3x}$

$-12x - 72 = 0$

$\underline{\quad +72 = +72}$

$$\frac{-12x}{-12} = \frac{72}{-12}$$

$x = -6$

2. $3x + 3 = x - 5$

$\underline{-x \qquad = -x}$

$2x + 3 = -5$

$\underline{\quad -3 = -3}$

$$\frac{2x}{2} = \frac{-8}{2}$$

$x = -4$

3. $2x - 11 = -8x + 109$

$\underline{+8x \qquad = +8x}$

$10x - 11 = 109$

$\underline{\quad +11 = +11}$

$$\frac{10x}{10} = \frac{120}{10}$$

$x = 12$

4. $6 - 8x = 20x + 20$

$\underline{\quad -20x = -20x}$

$6 - 28x = 20$

$\underline{-6 \qquad = -6}$

$$\frac{-28x}{-28} = \frac{14}{-28}$$

$x = -\dfrac{1}{2}$

5. $-x - 4 = -13x - 100$

$\underline{+13x \qquad = +13x}$

$12x - 4 = -100$

$\underline{\quad +4 = +4}$

$$\frac{12x}{12} = \frac{-96}{12}$$

$x = -8$

6. $3(k + 2) = 12k$

$3k + 6 = 12k$

$\underline{-12k \qquad = -12k}$

$-9k + 6 = 0$

$\underline{\quad -6 = -6}$

$$\frac{-9k}{-9} = \frac{-6}{-9}$$

$k = \dfrac{2}{3}$

7. $4y + 3 = 7\,(y + 1)$

$4y + 3 = 7y + 7$

$-7y\; = -7y$

$-3y + 3 = 7$

$-3 = -3$

$\dfrac{-3y}{-3} = \dfrac{4}{-3}$

$y = -\dfrac{4}{3}$

8. $2(x + 1) = \;3x - 1$

$2x + 2 = 3x - 1$

$-3x\; = -3x$

$-x + 2 = -1$

$+2 = -2$

$\dfrac{-x}{-1} = \dfrac{-3}{-1}$

$x = 3$

9. $3(a + 22) = 3(4a + 10)$

$3a + 66 = 12a + 30$

$-12a\; = -12a$

$-9a + 66 = 30$

$+66 = -66$

$\dfrac{-9a}{-9} = \dfrac{-36}{-9}$

$a = 4$

10. $5(z - 1) = 4(z + 4)$

$5z - 5 = 4z + 16$

$-4z\; = -4z$

$z - 5 = 16$

$+5 = +5$

$z = 21$

11. $6(y + 3) = 4(y + 9)$

$6y + 18 = 4y + 36$

$-4y\; = -4y$

$2y + 18 = 36$

$-18 = -18$

$\dfrac{2y}{2} = \dfrac{18}{2}$

$y = 9$

12. $7x - 6 - 9x = 12x - 48$

$-2x - 6 = 12x - 48$

$-12x\; = -12x$

$-14x - 6 = -48$

$+6 = +6$

$\dfrac{-14x}{-14} = \dfrac{-42}{-14}$

$x = 3$

13. $3x - x - 5 = x + 8$

$$2x - 5 = \cancel{x} + 8$$
$$-x \quad = \cancel{-x}$$
$$x - \cancel{5} = 8$$
$$\underline{+\cancel{5} = +5}$$
$$x = 13$$

14. $4x + 4 - 2x - x = 4x - 5$

$$x + 4 = \cancel{4x} - 5$$
$$-4x \quad = \cancel{-4x}$$
$$-3x + \cancel{4} = -5$$
$$\cancel{-4} = -4$$
$$\frac{1}{1}\frac{\cancel{-3}x}{\cancel{-3}} = \frac{\cancel{-9}^{3}}{\cancel{-3}_{1}}$$
$$x = 3$$

15. $6 + x - 2x + 3x - 4x = 3x + 4$

$$6 - 2x = \cancel{3x} + 4$$
$$-3x = \cancel{-3x}$$
$$\cancel{6} - 5x = 4$$
$$\cancel{-6} = -6$$
$$\frac{1}{1}\frac{\cancel{-5}x}{\cancel{-5}} = \frac{-2}{-5}$$
$$x = \frac{2}{5}$$

16. $5m - (m + 5) = 11$

$$5m - 1(m + 5) = 11$$
$$5m - 1m - 5 = 11$$
$$4m - \cancel{5} = 11$$
$$\underline{+\cancel{5} = +5}$$
$$\frac{1}{1}\frac{\cancel{4}m}{\cancel{4}} = \frac{\cancel{16}^{4}}{\cancel{4}_{1}}$$
$$m = 4$$

17. $y + 2(y - 3) = 4 - 2y$

$$y + 2y - 6 = 4 - 2y$$
$$3y - 6 = 4 - \cancel{2y}$$
$$+2y = \cancel{+2y}$$
$$5y - \cancel{6} = 4$$
$$\cancel{+6} = +6$$
$$\frac{1}{1}\frac{\cancel{5}y}{\cancel{5}} = \frac{\cancel{10}^{2}}{\cancel{5}_{1}}$$
$$y = 2$$

18. $-2(x - 4) - x = -x - 2$

$$-2x + 8 - x = -x - 2$$
$$-3x + 8 = \cancel{-x} - 2$$
$$+x \quad = \cancel{+x}$$
$$-2x + \cancel{8} = -2$$
$$\cancel{-8} = -8$$
$$\frac{1}{1}\frac{\cancel{-2}x}{\cancel{-2}} = \frac{\cancel{-10}^{5}}{\cancel{-2}_{1}}$$
$$x = 5$$

19. $2m - 3(m + 3) = -13(m + 1)$

$2m - 3m - 9 = -13m - 13$

$-m - 9 = -13m - 13$

$+13m \qquad = +13m$
———————————————
$12m - 9 = -13$

$ + 9 = +9$
———————————————
$\dfrac{^1\cancel{12}m}{_1\cancel{12}} = \dfrac{-\cancel{4}^1}{\cancel{12}_3}$

$m = -\dfrac{1}{3}$

20. $7y + 2(2y - 1) = -(4y + 5)$

$7y + 4y - 2 = -4y - 5$

$11y - 2 = -4y - 5$

$+4y \qquad = +4y$
———————————————
$15y - 2 = -5$

$ + 2 = +2$
———————————————
$\dfrac{^1\cancel{15}y}{_1\cancel{15}} = \dfrac{-\cancel{3}^1}{\cancel{15}_5}$

$y = -\dfrac{1}{5}$

6.5 Chapter Test for Equations

Section 6.1

1. $x + 4 = 9$

$ -4 = -4$
—————————
$x = 5$

2. $x - 17 = 35$

$ +17 = +17$
—————————
$x = 52$

3. $k + 91 = -22$

$ -91 = -91$
—————————
$k = -113$

4. $-36 = x - 12$

$x - 12 = -36$

$ +12 = +12$
—————————
$x = -24$

Section 6.2

5. $5r = -35$

$\dfrac{^1\cancel{5}r}{_1\cancel{5}} = \dfrac{-\cancel{35}^7}{\cancel{5}_1}$

$r = -7$

6. $-81 = -9x$

$\dfrac{^1\cancel{-9}x}{_1\cancel{-9}} = \dfrac{\cancel{-81}^9}{\cancel{-9}_1}$

$x = 9$

7. $\dfrac{x}{8} = -16$

$^1\cancel{8} \cdot \dfrac{x}{\cancel{8}_1} = -16 \cdot 8$

$x = -128$

8. $\dfrac{-4}{9}d = -20$

$\left(\dfrac{^1\cancel{-9}}{\cancel{4}}\right)\left(\dfrac{\cancel{-4}}{\cancel{9}_1}\right)^1 d = \dfrac{\cancel{-20}^5}{1}\left(\dfrac{-9}{\cancel{4}}\right)_1$

$d = 45$

Section 6.3

9. $5y - 4 = 26$

$$\underline{+ 4 = +4}$$

$$5y = 30$$

$$\frac{\overset{1}{\cancel{5}}y}{\underset{1}{\cancel{5}}} = \frac{\overset{6}{\cancel{30}}}{\underset{1}{\cancel{5}}}$$

$$y = 6$$

10. $\dfrac{-x}{4} + 6 = -14$

$$\underline{\quad -6 = -6}$$

$$\frac{-x}{4} = -20$$

$$\overset{1}{\cancel{4}} \cdot \frac{-x}{\underset{1}{\cancel{4}}} = -20 \cdot 4$$

$$-x = -80$$

$$\frac{\cancel{-x}}{\cancel{-1}} = \frac{-80}{-1}$$

$$x = 80$$

11. $2 = -3c - 10$

$$-3c - 10 = 2$$

$$\underline{\quad + 10 = +10}$$

$$-3c = 12$$

$$\frac{\overset{1}{\cancel{-3}}c}{\underset{1}{\cancel{-3}}} = \frac{\overset{4}{\cancel{12}}}{\underset{1}{\cancel{-3}}}$$

$$c = -4$$

12. $8 - \dfrac{1}{5}x = 5$

$$\underline{-8 \qquad\quad = -8}$$

$$-\frac{1}{5}x = -3$$

$$\left(\frac{\overset{1}{\cancel{-5}}}{1}\right)\left(-\frac{1}{\underset{1}{\cancel{5}}}\right)x = \frac{-3}{1}\left(\frac{5}{1}\right)$$

$$x = 15$$

Section 6.4

13. $9n - 15 = 6n$

$$\underline{-6n \qquad = -6n}$$

$$3n - 15 = 0$$

$$\underline{\quad + 15 = +15}$$

$$\frac{\overset{1}{\cancel{3}}n}{\underset{1}{\cancel{3}}} = \frac{\overset{5}{\cancel{15}}}{\cancel{3}}_1$$

$$n = 5$$

14. $4x - 9 = 7x - 12$

$$\underline{-7x \qquad = -7x}$$

$$-3x - 9 = -12$$

$$\underline{\quad + 9 = +9}$$

$$\frac{\overset{1}{\cancel{-3}}x}{\underset{1}{\cancel{-3}}} = \frac{\overset{1}{\cancel{-3}}}{\underset{1}{\cancel{-3}}}$$

$$x = 1$$

15. $6y - 3 = 3(y + 2)$

$6y - 3 = 3y + 6$

$-3y \quad = -3y$

$3y - 3 = 6$

$ +3 = +3$

$\dfrac{\cancel{3}^1 y}{\cancel{3}_1} = \dfrac{\cancel{9}^3}{\cancel{3}_1}$

$y = 3$

16. $5m - 2m + 4 = 3m + m - 1$

$3m + 4 = 4m - 1$

$-4m \quad = -4m$

$-m + 4 = -1$

$ -4 = -4$

$\dfrac{-m}{-1} = \dfrac{-5}{-1}$

$m = 5$

17. $5(3x + 6) = 3(x + 18)$

$15x + 30 = 3x + 54$

$-3x \quad = -3x$

$12x + 30 = 54$

$ -30 = -30$

$\dfrac{\cancel{12}^1 x}{\cancel{12}_1} = \dfrac{\cancel{24}^2}{\cancel{12}_1}$

$x = 2$

18. $-4x - 3 + 2x - 6 = -7x + 6$

$-2x - 9 = -7x + 6$

$+7x \quad = +7x$

$5x - 9 = 6$

$ +9 = +9$

$\dfrac{\cancel{5}^1 x}{\cancel{5}_1} = \dfrac{\cancel{15}^3}{\cancel{5}_1}$

$x = 3$

19. $x - 5 + 4x = 4(x - 3)$

$5x - 5 = 4x - 12$

$-4x \quad = -4x$

$x - 5 = -12$

$ +5 = +5$

$x = -7$

20. $2(y + 8) - 4 = 8y$

$2y + 16 - 4 = 8y$

$2y + 12 = 8y$

$-8y \quad = -8y$

$-6y + 12 = 0$

$ -12 = -12$

$\dfrac{\cancel{-6}^1 y}{\cancel{-6}_1} = \dfrac{\cancel{-12}^2}{\cancel{-6}_1}$

$y = 2$

Practice Test 1
Cumulative Skills Test

Section

(1.1) 1.
$$\overset{1\,1\ 1\,1}{57{,}942}$$
$$+\ 78{,}859$$
$$\overline{136{,}801}$$

(1.2) 2.
$$\overset{1\ 10}{\underset{}{\overset{0\ 12}{}}}\ \overset{9\ 10}{\underset{}{\overset{2\ \cancel{10}}{\cancel{2\,1{,}3}\,0\,0}}}$$
$$-\ 17{,}4\,5\,2$$
$$\overline{3{,}8\,4\,8}$$

(1.3) 3.
$$\overset{3\quad 3}{\underset{}{\overset{3\quad 3}{4{,}706}}}$$
$$\times\ 505$$
$$\overline{23\ 530}$$
$$\underline{2\ 353\ 00}$$
$$2{,}376{,}530$$

(1.4) 4.
$$\overset{2}{\underset{1}{530}}\overline{)\,25{,}075}\quad 47\,\text{r.}165$$
$$\underline{-21\ 20}$$
$$3\ 875$$
$$\underline{-3\ 710}$$
$$165$$

(2.1) 5. $39 = \dfrac{39}{1}$ in fraction form

(2.1) 6. $\dfrac{36}{5} = 5\overline{)36}\ \overset{7\frac{1}{5}}{}$ $7\dfrac{1}{5}$ is the mixed number.
$$\underline{-35}$$
$$1$$

(2.1) 7. $2\dfrac{3}{5} = \dfrac{\left(2 \overset{10}{\times} 5\right) + 3}{5} = \dfrac{13}{5}$

(2.1) 8. $\dfrac{1}{3}\quad \overset{\ 9\ \ 1}{\cancel{27}\,3}$
$$\dfrac{1}{3} = \dfrac{1}{3}$$
$$\text{yes}$$

(2.2) 9. $4 \times \dfrac{7}{9} = \dfrac{4}{1} \times \dfrac{7}{9} = \dfrac{28}{9} = 3\dfrac{1}{9}$

(2.2) 10. $4\dfrac{3}{5} \times 2\dfrac{1}{2} \times 1\dfrac{5}{23} = \dfrac{\cancel{23}}{\cancel{5}_1} \times \dfrac{\cancel{5}^1}{\cancel{2}_1} \times \dfrac{\cancel{28}^{14}}{\cancel{23}_1} = \dfrac{14}{1} = 14$

(2.3) 11. $\dfrac{5}{8} \div \dfrac{25}{16} = \dfrac{\cancel{5}^1}{\cancel{8}_1} \times \dfrac{\cancel{16}^2}{\cancel{25}_5} = \dfrac{2}{5}$

(2.3) 12. $\dfrac{3}{7} \div 2 = \dfrac{3}{7} \div \dfrac{2}{1} = \dfrac{3}{7} \times \dfrac{1}{2} = \dfrac{3}{14}$

(2.3) 13. $4\dfrac{4}{5} \div \dfrac{8}{3} = \dfrac{24}{5} \div \dfrac{8}{3} = \dfrac{\overset{3}{\cancel{24}}}{5} \times \dfrac{3}{\underset{1}{\cancel{8}}} = \dfrac{9}{5} = 1\dfrac{4}{5}$

(2.4) 14. $\lfloor 7 \ \ 4$ LCD = 7 • 4 = 28

(2.4) 15.

$7\lfloor 21 \ \ 35$

$\quad \quad 3 \ \ 5$ LCD = 7 • 3 • 5 = 105

(2.4) 16.

$2\lfloor 15 \ \ 12 \ \ 8$ LCD = 2 • 2 • 3 • 5 • 1 • 2 = 120

$2\lfloor 15 \ \ 6 \ \ 4$

$3\lfloor 15 \ \ 3 \ \ 2$

$\quad \quad 5 \ \ 1 \ \ 2$

(2.5) 17.

$3\lfloor 5 \ \ 3 \ \ 15$

$5\lfloor 5 \ \ 1 \ \ 5$

$\quad \ 1 \ \ 1 \ \ 1$

LCD = 3 • 5 • 1 • 1 • 1 = 15

$2\dfrac{3}{5} \cdot \dfrac{3}{3} = \quad 2\dfrac{9}{15}$

$\dfrac{1}{3} \cdot \dfrac{5}{5} = \quad \dfrac{5}{15}$

$+ \ 6\dfrac{2}{15} \quad = + \ 6\dfrac{2}{15}$

$\quad\quad\quad\quad\quad\quad 8\dfrac{16}{15}$

$\dfrac{16}{15} = 1\dfrac{1}{15}$

$8 + 1\dfrac{1}{15} = 9\dfrac{1}{15}$

(2.6) 18.

$2\lfloor 88 \ \ 44$

$2\lfloor 44 \ \ 22$

$11\lfloor 22 \ \ 11$

$\quad \ 2 \ \ 1$

LCD = 2 • 2 • 11 • 2 • 1 = 22

$\dfrac{53}{88} \quad\quad = \quad \dfrac{53}{88}$

$- \ \dfrac{19}{44} \cdot \dfrac{2}{2} = - \dfrac{38}{88}$

$\quad\quad\quad\quad\quad\quad \dfrac{15}{88}$

(2.6) 19.

$2\lfloor 4 \ \ 6$

$\quad \ 2 \ \ 3$

LCD = 2 • 2 • 3 = 12

$26\dfrac{1}{4} \cdot \dfrac{3}{3} = 2\overset{5\frac{12}{12}}{\cancel{6}}\dfrac{3}{12} = 25\dfrac{15}{12}$

$- \ 5\dfrac{5}{6} \cdot \dfrac{2}{2} \ - \ 5\dfrac{10}{12} = -5\dfrac{10}{12}$

$\quad\quad\quad\quad\quad\quad\quad 20\dfrac{5}{12}$

(3.1) 20. 9   **(3.1)** 21. 0.0067   **(3.1)** 22. 0.0206

(3.2) 23. 346.7⑧5 = 346.79   **(3.2)** 24. 87,9④3 = 87,940

(3.3) 25.
```
    4.2300
    1.5000
  + 7.2341
   12.9641
```

(3.3) 26.
```
   2 14
  23.479
 −0.960
  22.519
```

(3.4) 27.
```
        1
        2
        5
     0.171
   × 0.238
     1 368
    1 5 13
    34 2
  0.040 698
```

(3.5) 28.
```
        30. = 30
  0.02)0.60.
        -6
        00
```

(3.5) 29.
```
    2    22.④5 = 22.5
    1
  24)539. 0 0
     -48
      59
     -48
      110
      -96
      140
     -120
       20
```

(3.6) 30. $0.25 = \dfrac{\overset{1}{\cancel{25}}}{\underset{4}{\cancel{100}}} = \dfrac{1}{4}$

(3.6) 31.
```
      0.75
  4)3.00
   -2 8
     20
    -20
      0
```

(3.7) 32.
a. 0.20   b. 0.02
     0.02   0.20
     0.30   0.30
     0.33   0.33

c. 0.02   0.2   0.3   0.33

(3.7) 33.
a. $\dfrac{1}{5} =$
```
      0.2
  5)1.0
   -1 0
      0
```
b. 0.27 > 0.20

c. 0.27 > $\dfrac{1}{5}$

(3.7) 34.
a.
```
  3|5 15 30
  5|5  5 10
    1  1  2
```
LCD = 3 • 5 • 1 • 1 • 2 = 30

b. $\dfrac{3}{5} = \dfrac{18}{30}$

    $\dfrac{7}{15} = \dfrac{14}{30}$

    $\dfrac{11}{30} = \dfrac{11}{30}$

c. $\dfrac{11}{30} \quad \dfrac{14}{30} \quad \dfrac{18}{30}$

d. $\dfrac{11}{30} \quad \dfrac{7}{15} \quad \dfrac{3}{5}$

(4.1) 35. $\dfrac{25}{4} = \dfrac{n}{12}$

$$\dfrac{\cancel{4}^{1}\,n}{\cancel{4}_{1}} = \dfrac{\cancel{300}^{75}}{\cancel{4}_{1}\cancel{2}_{1}}$$

$n = 75$

(4.2) 36. $\dfrac{40}{16} = \dfrac{x}{100}$

$$\dfrac{\cancel{16}^{1}\,x}{\cancel{16}_{1}} = \dfrac{4{,}000}{16}$$

$x = 250\%$

(4.2) 37. $\dfrac{x}{90} = \dfrac{30}{100}$

$$\dfrac{\cancel{100}^{1}\,x}{\cancel{100}_{1}} = \dfrac{2{,}700}{100}$$

$x = 27$

(4.2) 38. $\dfrac{50}{x} = \dfrac{20}{100}$

$$\dfrac{\cancel{20}\,x}{\cancel{20}} = \dfrac{5{,}000}{20}$$

$x = 250$

(4.2) 39. Change $12\dfrac{1}{2}$ to an improper fraction. $12\dfrac{1}{2} = \dfrac{25}{2}$

$$\dfrac{15}{x} = \dfrac{\frac{25}{2}}{100}$$

$$\dfrac{25}{2}x = 15\,(100)$$

$$\dfrac{\cancel{2}^{1}}{\cancel{25}_{1}} \cdot \dfrac{\cancel{25}^{1}}{\cancel{2}_{1}}\,x = \dfrac{\cancel{1{,}500}^{60}}{1} \cdot \dfrac{2}{\cancel{25}_{1}}$$

$$x = 120$$

(4.2) 40. $$\dfrac{\frac{3}{16}}{\frac{3}{4}} = \dfrac{x}{100}$$

$$\dfrac{3}{4}x = \dfrac{3}{16}\,(100)$$

$$\dfrac{\cancel{4}^{1}}{\cancel{3}_{1}} \cdot \dfrac{\cancel{3}^{1}}{\cancel{4}_{1}}\,x = \dfrac{\cancel{3}^{1}}{\cancel{16}_{\,4}} \cdot \dfrac{\cancel{100}^{25}}{1} \cdot \dfrac{\cancel{4}^{1}}{\cancel{3}_{1}}$$

$$x = 25\%$$

(4.3) 41. $12.5\% = \dfrac{12.5}{100} \cdot \dfrac{10}{10} = \dfrac{\cancel{125}^{5\;1}}{\cancel{1000}_{\,40\;8}} = \dfrac{1}{8}$

(4.3) 42.
$$\frac{6}{18} = \frac{x}{100}$$
$$18x = 6(100)$$
$$\frac{\cancel{18}x}{\cancel{18}} = \frac{600}{18}$$
$$x = 33.3\% \text{ or } 33\frac{1}{3}\%$$

(4.3) 43. 6 : 20
$$\frac{6}{20} = \frac{x}{100}$$
$$20x = 6(100)$$
$$\frac{\cancel{20}x}{\cancel{20}} = \frac{600}{20}$$
$$x = 30\%$$

(4.4) 44.
$$\frac{6.5}{20\%} = \frac{6.5}{0.20} = \frac{6.5}{0.2} = 32.5$$

$$
\begin{array}{r}
3\,2.5 \\
0.2\overline{)6.5.0} \\
\underline{-6} \\
0\,5 \\
\underline{-4} \\
1\,0 \\
\underline{-1\,0} \\
0
\end{array}
$$

(4.4) 45. $66\% = 66. = 0.66$

(4.4) 46. $0.456 = 45.6\%$

(5.1) 47. $(-17) + (-4)$
-21

Negative + negative = negative.

(5.1) 48. $25 + (-8)$
17

a. Subtract $25 - 8 = 17$.
b. Larger number 25 is positive.
c. The answer is $+17$.

(5.1) 49. $-36 + 36$
0

Any number + its opposite = 0.

(5.1) 50. $-18 + 10$
-8

a. Subtract $18 - 10 = 8$.
b. Larger number 18 is negative.
c. The answer is -8.

(5.2) 51. $13 - 15$
$13 + (-15)$
-2

(5.2) 52. $-8 - 19$
$-8 + (-19)$
-27

(5.2) 53. $-5 - (-23)$
$-5 + 23$
18

(5.2) 54. $7 - (-4)$
$7 + 4$
11

(5.3) 55. $(-9)(-10) = 90$

(5.3) 56. $(4)(-17) = -68$

(5.3) 57. $\dfrac{\cancel{81}^{9}}{\cancel{9}_{1}} = 9$

(5.3) 58. $\dfrac{\overset{1}{-\cancel{15}}}{_{4}\cancel{60}} = \dfrac{-1}{4}$

(5.4) 59. $7x - 3x + 12x$
$4x + 12x$
$16x$

(5.4) 60. $5xy^2 - 3xy - xy$
$5xy^2 - 4xy$

(5.5) 61. $(x^2 - 2) - (3x^2 - 4x + 5)$
$(x^2 - 2) - 1(3x^2 - 4x + 5)$
$x^2 \,\underset{}{(-2)} - 3x^2 + 4x \,(-5)$
$-2x^2 - 7 + 4x$

(5.5) 62. $7(r + 6)$
$7r + 42$

(5.5) 63. $-3(x^2 + 7x - 9)$
$-3x^2 - 21x + 27$

(5.5) 64. $-(a - 10)$
$-1(a - 10)$
$-1a + 10$
$-a + 10$

(6.1) 65. $x + \cancel{37} = -26$
$\underline{-\cancel{37} = -37}$
$x = -63$

(6.1) 66. $x - \cancel{71} = 23$
$\underline{+\cancel{71} = +71}$
$x = 94$

(6.2) 67. $-5x = -80$
$\dfrac{^{1}\cancel{-5}x}{_{1}\cancel{-5}} = \dfrac{\cancel{-80}^{16}}{\cancel{-5}_{1}}$
$x = 16$

(6.2) 68. $\dfrac{2}{5}x = -14$
$\dfrac{^{1}\cancel{5}}{_{1}\cancel{2}} \cdot \dfrac{\cancel{2}^{1}}{\cancel{5}_{1}} x = \dfrac{-\cancel{14}^{7}}{1} \cdot \dfrac{5}{\cancel{2}_{1}}$
$x = -35$

(6.3) 69. $3x + \cancel{7} = 22$
$\underline{-\cancel{7} = -7}$
$3x = 15$
$\dfrac{^{1}\cancel{3}x}{_{1}\cancel{3}} = \dfrac{\cancel{15}^{5}}{\cancel{3}_{1}}$
$x = 5$

(6.3) 70.

$$\cancel{13} - \frac{3x}{2} = 37$$

$$\underline{\cancel{13} \qquad\quad = -13}$$

$$-\frac{3x}{2} = 24$$

$$\,^1\!\left(-\frac{\cancel{2}}{\cancel{3}}\right)\!\left(-\frac{\cancel{3}x}{\cancel{2}}\right)^1_1 = \frac{^8\cancel{24}}{1}\left(-\frac{2}{\cancel{3}}\right)_1$$

$$x = -16$$

(6.4) 71.

$$3x - 10 = \cancel{-9x}$$

$$\underline{+9x \qquad = \cancel{+9x}}$$

$$12x \cancel{-10} = 0$$

$$\underline{\qquad \cancel{+10} = +10}$$

$$\frac{^1\cancel{12}x}{_1\cancel{12}} = \frac{\cancel{10}^5}{\cancel{12}_6}$$

$$x = \frac{5}{6}$$

(6.4) 72.

$$2(x + 1) = 3x - 1$$

$$2x + 2 = \cancel{3x} - 1$$

$$\underline{-3x \qquad = \cancel{-3x}}$$

$$-x \cancel{+2} = -1$$

$$\underline{\cancel{-2} = -2}$$

$$\frac{-x}{-1} = \frac{-3}{-1}$$

$$x = 3$$

(6.4) 73.

$$2(y + 3) = 4(y - 6)$$

$$2y + 6 = \cancel{4y} - 24$$

$$\underline{-4y \qquad = \cancel{-4y}}$$

$$-2y \cancel{+6} = -24$$

$$\underline{\cancel{-6} = -6}$$

$$\frac{^1\cancel{-2}y}{_1\cancel{-2}} = \frac{\cancel{-30}^{15}}{\cancel{-2}_1}$$

$$y = 15$$

(6.4) 74.

$$3(x + 3) + 5 = 2x$$

$$3x + 9 + 5 = 2x$$

$$3x + 14 = 2x$$

$$\underline{-2x \qquad = -2x}$$

$$x \cancel{+14} = 0$$

$$\underline{\cancel{-14} = -14}$$

$$x = -14$$

(6.4) 75.

$$13 + 5x - 7 = 3x - 8 - 12x$$

$$6 + 5x = \cancel{-9x} - 8$$

$$\underline{+ 9x = \cancel{+9x}}$$

$$\cancel{6} + 14x = -8$$

$$\underline{\cancel{-6} \qquad = -6}$$

$$\frac{^1\cancel{14}x}{_1\cancel{14}} = \frac{-\cancel{14}^1}{\cancel{14}_1}$$

$$x = -1$$

Practice Test 2
Combined Skills Test

Section

(3.1) 1. $\dfrac{47}{100,000}$ = 0.00047

(3.1) 2. 1,346.9<u>79</u>

(3.1) 3. 16.04

(3.2) 4. 5,642.01⑧2 =
5,642.018

(3.3) 5.
$$\begin{array}{r} 9.6\mathbf{00} \\ 8.234 \\ + 1.05\mathbf{0} \\ \hline 18.884 \end{array}$$

(3.3) 6.
$$\begin{array}{r} \overset{9\ 12}{\cancel{3}\ \cancel{10}}\overset{2\ 10}{}\overset{9\ 10}{} \\ \overset{0\ \cancel{10}}{4\,0\,\cancel{3}.\cancel{1}\,0\,0} \\ -\ 1\,5\,.\,2\,3\,6 \\ \hline 3\,8\,7\,.\,8\,6\,4 \end{array}$$

(3.4) 7.
$$\begin{array}{r} \overset{1\ 1}{14.56} \\ \times\ 0.2 \\ \hline 2.912 \end{array}$$

(3.5) 8.
$$\begin{array}{r} 2.1 \\ 0.43\overline{)0.90.3} \\ -86 \\ \hline 4\,3 \\ -4\,3 \\ \hline 0 \end{array}$$

(2.1) 9. $\dfrac{\cancel{25}^{\,1}}{300_{\,12}} = \dfrac{1}{12}$

(2.1) 10. $\dfrac{50}{7} = 7\dfrac{1}{7}$
$$\begin{array}{r} 7\frac{1}{7} \\ 7\overline{)50} \\ -49 \\ \hline 1 \end{array}$$

(2.1) 11. $\dfrac{2}{5}\qquad\dfrac{8}{25}$

$\dfrac{2}{5} \ne \dfrac{8}{25}$

no

(2.4) and **(2.5)** 12.

$$\begin{array}{r|ccc} 2 & 4 & 6 & 12 \\ 2 & 2 & 3 & 6 \\ 3 & 1 & 3 & 3 \\ \hline & 1 & 1 & 1 \end{array}$$

LCD = 2 • 2 • 3 • 1 • 1 • 1 = 12

$1\dfrac{1}{4} \bullet \dfrac{3}{3} = 1\dfrac{3}{12}$

$2\dfrac{5}{6} \bullet \dfrac{2}{2} = 2\dfrac{10}{12}$

$+\dfrac{1}{12} \qquad = +\dfrac{1}{12}$

$\overline{3\dfrac{14}{12}}$

$\dfrac{14}{12} = 1\dfrac{2}{12} = 1\dfrac{1}{6}$

$3 + 1\dfrac{1}{6} = 4\dfrac{1}{6}$

(2.4) and **(2.6)** 13.

$$\underline{|5 \quad 7}$$

$$\text{LCD} = 5 \cdot 7 = 35$$

$$37\frac{1}{5} \cdot \frac{7}{7} = 37\frac{7}{35} = \overset{216}{36}\frac{\overset{42}{}}{35} \quad \overset{6\frac{35}{35}}{}$$

$$-9\frac{4}{7} \cdot \frac{5}{5} = -9\frac{20}{35} = -9\frac{20}{35}$$

$$\overline{}$$

$$27\frac{22}{35}$$

(2.2) 14. $1\frac{3}{4} \times 2\frac{2}{3} \times 1\frac{4}{5} = \frac{7}{{}_1\cancel{4}} \times \frac{\cancel{8}^2}{\cancel{3}_1} \times \frac{\cancel{9}^3}{5} = \frac{42}{5} = 8\frac{2}{5}$

(2.3) 15. $\frac{5}{9} \div 1\frac{1}{3} = \frac{5}{9} \div \frac{4}{3} = \frac{5}{{}_3\cancel{9}} \times \frac{\cancel{3}^1}{4} = \frac{5}{12}$

(4.3) 16. $62.5\% = \frac{62.5}{100} \cdot \frac{10}{10} = \frac{\cancel{625}}{\cancel{1000}} = \frac{5}{8}$

(3.6) 17. $\frac{1}{8}$ =

$$8\overline{)1.000}\ ^{\;0.125}$$
$$\underline{-8}$$
$$20$$
$$\underline{-16}$$
$$40$$
$$\underline{-40}$$
$$0$$

(4.4) 18. $650\% = 6.5\cancel{0} = 6.5$

(4.4) 19. $\frac{49}{7} = 7.00 = 700\%$

(4.2) 20. $4 : 20 = \frac{4}{20}$

$$\frac{4}{20} = \frac{x}{100}$$

$$\frac{{}^1\cancel{20}x}{\cancel{20}_1} = \frac{400}{20}$$

$$x = 20\%$$

(4.4) 21. $0.017 = 1.7\%$

(3.6) 22. $\dfrac{13.4}{40\%} = \dfrac{13.4}{0.40} = \dfrac{13.4}{0.4} = 33.5$

$$0.4\overline{)13.4.0}\quad 3\ 3.5$$

$$\begin{array}{r} 3\ 3.5 \\ 0.4\,)\overline{13.4.0} \\ \underline{-12} \\ 1\ 4 \\ \underline{-1\ 2} \\ 2\ 0 \\ \underline{-2\ 0} \\ 0 \end{array}$$

(4.2) 23. $\dfrac{x}{72} = \dfrac{16.5}{100}$

$\dfrac{\cancel{100}x}{\cancel{100}} = \dfrac{1,188}{100}$

$x = 11.88$

(4.2) 24. Change $33\frac{1}{3}$ to an improper fraction.

$33\frac{1}{3} = \dfrac{100}{3}$

$\dfrac{45}{x} = \dfrac{\frac{100}{3}}{100}$

$\dfrac{100}{3}x = 4{,}500$

$\dfrac{\cancel{3}^{1}}{\cancel{100}_{1}} \cdot \dfrac{\cancel{100}^{1}}{\cancel{3}_{1}}\, x = \dfrac{\cancel{4{,}500}^{45}}{1} \cdot \dfrac{3}{\cancel{100}_{1}}$

$x = 135$

(4.2) 25. $\dfrac{210}{x} = \dfrac{35}{100}$

$\dfrac{\cancel{35}x}{\cancel{35}} = \dfrac{21{,}000}{35}$

$x = 600$

(4.2) 26. $\dfrac{\frac{1}{2}}{\frac{4}{5}} = \dfrac{x}{100}$

$\dfrac{4}{5}x = \dfrac{1}{2} \cdot 100$

$\dfrac{\cancel{5}^{1}}{\cancel{4}_{1}} \cdot \dfrac{\cancel{4}^{1}}{\cancel{5}_{1}}\, x = \dfrac{1}{\cancel{2}_{1}} \cdot \dfrac{\cancel{100}^{50\ 25}}{1} \cdot \dfrac{5}{\cancel{4}_{2}}$

$x = \dfrac{125}{2} = 62\frac{1}{2}\%$

OR Change to Decimals

$\dfrac{1}{2} = 0.5 \qquad \dfrac{4}{5} = 0.8$

$\dfrac{0.5}{0.8} = \dfrac{x}{100}$

$\dfrac{\cancel{0.8}x}{\cancel{0.8}} = \dfrac{50}{0.8}$

$x = 62.5\%$

(5.4) 27. $(x^2 - 5) - (-4x^2 + 5x - 1)$

$(x^2 - 5) - 1(-4x^2 + 5x - 1)$

$x^2 \boxed{-5} + 4x^2 - 5x \boxed{+1}$

$5x^2 - 4 - 5x$

(6.1) 28.　$-2v + 4 = -8$

$$\underline{\quad -4 = -4\quad}$$

$$\frac{^1\cancel{-2}\,v}{_1\cancel{-2}} = \frac{\cancel{-12}^{\,6}}{\cancel{-2}_{\,1}}$$

$$v = 6$$

(6.4) 29.　$5m + 8 = \overset{\frown}{3(m + 4)}$

$$5m + 8 = 3m + 12$$

$$\underline{-3m \quad\;\; = -3m\quad}$$

$$2m + 8 = 12$$

$$\underline{\quad -8 = -8\quad}$$

$$\frac{^1\cancel{2}\,m}{_1\cancel{2}} = \frac{\cancel{4}^{\,2}}{\cancel{2}_{\,1}}$$

$$m = 2$$

(6.4) 30.　$\overset{\frown}{4(x - 9)} + 12 = \overset{\frown}{-2(x - 6)}$

$$4x - 36 + 12 = -2x + 12$$

$$4x - 24 = -2x + 12$$

$$\underline{+2x \qquad\quad = +2x\quad}$$

$$6x - 24 = 12$$

$$\underline{\quad +24 = +24\quad}$$

$$\frac{^1\cancel{6}\,x}{_1\cancel{6}} = \frac{\cancel{36}^{\,6}}{\cancel{6}_{\,1}}$$

$$x = 6$$

(3.7) 31.　a.　0.570　　b.　0.500
　　　　　0.507　　　　0.507
　　　　　0.572　　　　0.570
　　　　　0.500　　　　0.572

　　c.　0.5　0.507　0.57　0.572

(3.7) 32.　a.　$\dfrac{3}{8} = $

$$\begin{array}{r} 0.375 \\ 8\overline{)3.000} \\ \underline{-2\;4} \\ 60 \\ \underline{-56} \\ 40 \\ \underline{-40} \\ 0 \end{array}$$

　　b. $0.350 < 0.375$

　　c. $0.35 < \dfrac{3}{8}$

(3.7) 33.　a.

$$\begin{array}{c|ccc} 2 & 8 & 4 & 6 \\ \hline 2 & 4 & 2 & 3 \\ \hline & 2 & 1 & 3 \end{array}$$

$$\text{LCD} = 2 \bullet 2 \bullet 1 \bullet 3 = 24$$

　　b. $\dfrac{1}{8} = \dfrac{3}{24}$　　c. $\dfrac{3}{24}\ \dfrac{4}{24}\ \dfrac{6}{24}$

　　　$\dfrac{1}{4} = \dfrac{6}{24}$　　d. $\dfrac{1}{8}\ \dfrac{1}{6}\ \dfrac{1}{4}$

　　　$\dfrac{1}{6} = \dfrac{4}{24}$

7.0 Pretest for Household Measures

Sections 7.1 and 7.2

1. $\dfrac{\overset{5}{\cancel{40}}\text{ oz.}}{1} \cdot \dfrac{1\text{ lb.}}{\underset{2}{\cancel{16}}\text{ oz.}} = \dfrac{5}{2} = 2\dfrac{1}{2}\text{ pounds}$

2. $\dfrac{4\text{ ft.}}{1} \cdot \dfrac{12\text{ in.}}{1\text{ ft.}} = 48\text{ inches}$

3. $\dfrac{3\text{ pt.}}{1} \cdot \dfrac{1\text{ qt.}}{2\text{ pt.}} = \dfrac{3}{2} = 1\dfrac{1}{2}\text{ quarts}$

4. $\dfrac{\overset{5}{\cancel{15}}\text{ tsp.}}{1} \cdot \dfrac{1\text{ T}}{\underset{1}{\cancel{3}}\text{ tsp.}} = 5\text{ tablespoons}$

5. $\dfrac{25\text{ ft.}}{1} \cdot \dfrac{1\text{ yd.}}{3\text{ ft.}} = \dfrac{25}{3} = 8\dfrac{1}{3}\text{ yards}$

6. $\dfrac{\overset{3}{\cancel{6}}\text{ T.}}{1} \cdot \dfrac{1\text{ fl. oz.}}{\underset{1}{\cancel{2}}\text{ T.}} = 3\text{ fluid ounces}$

7. $\dfrac{\overset{5}{\cancel{5,000}}\text{ lbs.}}{1} \cdot \dfrac{1\text{ ton}}{\underset{2}{\cancel{2,000}}\text{ lbs.}} = \dfrac{5}{2} = 2\dfrac{1}{2}\text{ tons}$

8. $\dfrac{17\text{ mi.}}{1} \cdot \dfrac{5,280\text{ ft.}}{1\text{ mi.}} = 89,760\text{ feet}$

Section 7.3

9. $\dfrac{3\text{ cups}}{1} \cdot \dfrac{8\text{ fl. oz.}}{1\text{ cup}} \cdot \dfrac{2\text{ T.}}{1\text{ fl. oz.}} = 48\text{ tablespoons}$

10. $\dfrac{\overset{1}{\cancel{8}}\text{ pt.}}{1} \cdot \dfrac{1\text{ qt.}}{\underset{1}{\cancel{2}}\text{ pt.}} \cdot \dfrac{1\text{ gal.}}{\underset{1}{\cancel{4}}\text{ qt.}} = 1\text{ gallon}$

7.1 Practice Length Conversions

1. $\dfrac{9 \cancel{\text{ft.}}}{1} \cdot \dfrac{12\,\text{in.}}{1 \cancel{\text{ft.}}} = 108 \text{ inches}$

2. $\dfrac{\overset{6}{\cancel{72}} \text{ in.}}{1} \cdot \dfrac{1\,\text{ft.}}{\underset{1}{\cancel{12}} \text{ in.}} = 6\,\text{feet}$

3. $\dfrac{4 \cancel{\text{ mi.}}}{1} \cdot \dfrac{5{,}280\,\text{ft.}}{1 \cancel{\text{ mi.}}} = 21{,}120\,\text{feet}$

4. $\dfrac{\overset{2}{\cancel{6}}\text{ ft.}}{1} \cdot \dfrac{1\,\text{yd.}}{\underset{1}{\cancel{3}}\,\cancel{\text{ft.}}} = 2\,\text{yards}$

5. $\dfrac{\overset{924}{\cancel{9{,}240}}\text{ ft.}}{1} \cdot \dfrac{1\,\text{mi.}}{\underset{528}{\cancel{5{,}280}}\,\cancel{\text{ft.}}} = \dfrac{924}{528} = 1.75 \text{ miles}$

6. $\dfrac{430 \cancel{\text{ ft.}}}{1} \cdot \dfrac{1\,\text{yd.}}{3 \cancel{\text{ft.}}} = \dfrac{430}{3} = 143\tfrac{1}{3}\,\text{yards}$

7. $\dfrac{\overset{10}{\cancel{120}} \text{ in.}}{1} \cdot \dfrac{1 \cancel{\text{ft.}}}{\underset{1}{\cancel{12}} \text{ in.}} = 10\,\text{feet}$

8. $\dfrac{18 \cancel{\text{ mi.}}}{1} \cdot \dfrac{5{,}280\,\text{ft.}}{1 \cancel{\text{ mi.}}} = 95{,}040\,\text{feet}$

9. $\dfrac{42 \cancel{\text{ ft.}}}{1} \cdot \dfrac{12\,\text{in.}}{1 \cancel{\text{ ft.}}} = 504\,\text{inches}$

10. $\dfrac{\overset{11}{\cancel{33}} \cancel{\text{ ft.}}}{1} \cdot \dfrac{1\,\text{yd.}}{\underset{1}{\cancel{3}} \cancel{\text{ft.}}} = 11\,\text{yards}$

11. $\dfrac{720 \cancel{\text{ yd.}}}{1} \cdot \dfrac{3\,\text{ft.}}{1 \cancel{\text{ yd.}}} = 2{,}160\,\text{feet}$

12. $\dfrac{\overset{792}{\cancel{7{,}920}} \text{ ft.}}{1} \cdot \dfrac{1\,\text{mi.}}{\underset{528}{\cancel{5{,}280}} \text{ ft.}} = \dfrac{792}{528} = 1.5 \text{ miles}$

13. $\dfrac{30 \text{ ft.}}{1} \cdot \dfrac{12 \text{ in.}}{1 \text{ ft.}} = 360 \text{ inches}$

14. $\dfrac{\overset{231}{\cancel{693}} \text{ ft.}}{1} \cdot \dfrac{1 \text{ yd.}}{\underset{1}{\cancel{3}} \text{ ft.}} = 231 \text{ yards}$

15. $\dfrac{\overset{5}{\cancel{30}} \text{ in.}}{1} \cdot \dfrac{1 \text{ ft.}}{\underset{2}{\cancel{12}} \text{ in.}} = \dfrac{5}{2} = 2\dfrac{1}{2} \text{ feet}$

16. $\dfrac{10 \text{ mi.}}{1} \cdot \dfrac{5{,}280 \text{ ft.}}{1 \text{ mi.}} = 52{,}800 \text{ feet}$

17. $\dfrac{\overset{2{,}772}{\cancel{27{,}720}} \text{ ft.}}{1} \cdot \dfrac{1 \text{ mi.}}{\underset{528}{\cancel{5{,}280}} \text{ ft.}} = \dfrac{2{,}772}{528} = 5.25 \text{ miles}$

18. $\dfrac{29 \text{ yd.}}{1} \cdot \dfrac{3 \text{ ft.}}{1 \text{ yd.}} = 87 \text{ feet}$

19. $\dfrac{10 \text{ ft.}}{1} \cdot \dfrac{1 \text{ yd.}}{3 \text{ ft.}} = \dfrac{10}{3} = 3\dfrac{1}{3} \text{ yards}$

20. $\dfrac{1.25 \text{ mi.}}{1} \cdot \dfrac{5{,}280 \text{ ft.}}{1 \text{ mi.}} = 6{,}600 \text{ feet}$

7.2 Practice Weight Conversions

1. $\dfrac{\overset{2}{\cancel{32}} \text{ oz.}}{1} \cdot \dfrac{1 \text{ lb.}}{\underset{1}{\cancel{16}} \text{ oz.}} = 2 \text{ pounds}$

2. $\dfrac{3 \text{ lb.}}{1} \cdot \dfrac{16 \text{ oz.}}{1 \text{ lb.}} = 48 \text{ ounces}$

3. $\dfrac{2.5 \text{ tons}}{1} \cdot \dfrac{2,000 \text{ lb.}}{1 \text{ ton}} = 5,000 \text{ pounds}$

4. $\dfrac{\overset{5}{\cancel{\underset{}{2,500}}}\text{ lb.}}{1} \cdot \dfrac{1 \text{ ton}}{\underset{4}{\overset{20}{\cancel{2,000}}} \text{ lb.}} = \dfrac{5}{4} = 1.25 \text{ tons}$

5. $5\dfrac{1}{4} \text{ lb.} = 5.25 \text{ lb.} \qquad \dfrac{5.25 \text{ lb.}}{1} \cdot \dfrac{16 \text{ oz.}}{1 \text{ lb.}} = 84 \text{ ounces}$

6. $\dfrac{3}{4} \text{ ton} = 0.75 \text{ ton} \qquad \dfrac{0.75 \text{ ton}}{1} \cdot \dfrac{2,000 \text{ lb.}}{1 \text{ ton}} = 1,500 \text{ pounds}$

7. $\dfrac{\overset{3}{\cancel{12}} \text{ oz.}}{1} \cdot \dfrac{1 \text{ lb.}}{\underset{4}{\cancel{16}} \text{ oz.}} = \dfrac{3}{4} = 0.75 \text{ pound}$

8. $\dfrac{\overset{9}{\cancel{36}}\,3,600 \text{ lb.}}{1} \cdot \dfrac{1 \text{ ton}}{\underset{5}{\overset{20}{\cancel{2,000}}} \text{ lb.}} = \dfrac{9}{5} = 1\dfrac{4}{5} \text{ tons}$

9. $\dfrac{\overset{17}{\cancel{68}} \text{ oz.}}{1} \cdot \dfrac{1 \text{ lb.}}{\underset{4}{\cancel{16}} \text{ oz.}} = \dfrac{17}{4} = 4\dfrac{1}{4} \text{ pounds}$

10. $1\dfrac{1}{4} \text{ lb.} = 1.25 \text{ lb.} \qquad \dfrac{1.25 \text{ lb.}}{1} \cdot \dfrac{16 \text{ oz.}}{1 \text{ lb.}} = 20 \text{ ounces}$

11. $\dfrac{4 \text{ tons}}{1} \cdot \dfrac{2,000 \text{ lb.}}{1 \text{ ton}} = 8,000 \text{ pounds}$

12. $\dfrac{\overset{10}{\cancel{20,000}} \text{ lb.}}{1} \cdot \dfrac{1 \text{ ton}}{\underset{1}{\cancel{2,000}} \text{ lb.}} = 10 \text{ tons}$

13. $\dfrac{\overset{9}{\cancel{36}}\,144 \text{ oz.}}{1} \cdot \dfrac{1 \text{ lb.}}{\underset{1}{\overset{4}{\cancel{16}}} \text{ oz.}} = 9 \text{ pounds}$

14. $\dfrac{\overset{15}{\cancel{15,000}} \text{ lb.}}{1} \cdot \dfrac{1 \text{ ton}}{\underset{2}{\cancel{2,000}} \text{ lb.}} = \dfrac{15}{2} = 7\dfrac{1}{2}$ tons

15. $\dfrac{\overset{1}{\cancel{16}} \text{ oz.}}{1} \cdot \dfrac{1 \text{ lb.}}{\underset{1}{\cancel{16}} \text{ oz.}} = 1 \text{ pound}$

16. $1\dfrac{1}{2}$ tons $= 1.5$ tons $\qquad \dfrac{1.5 \cancel{\text{ tons}}}{1} \cdot \dfrac{2,000 \text{ lb.}}{1 \cancel{\text{ ton}}} = 3,000 \text{ pounds}$

17. $\dfrac{\overset{7}{\cancel{\overset{28}{\cancel{112}}}} \text{ oz.}}{1} \cdot \dfrac{1 \text{ lb.}}{\underset{1}{\overset{4}{\cancel{16}}} \text{ oz.}} = 7 \text{ pounds}$

18. $\dfrac{\overset{1}{\cancel{1,000}} \text{ lb.}}{1} \cdot \dfrac{1 \text{ ton}}{\underset{2}{\cancel{2,000}} \text{ lb.}} = \dfrac{1}{2} \text{ ton}$

19. $\dfrac{16 \cancel{\text{ tons}}}{1} \cdot \dfrac{2,000 \text{ lb.}}{1 \cancel{\text{ ton}}} = 32,000 \text{ pounds}$

20. $\dfrac{5.5 \cancel{\text{ lb.}}}{1} \cdot \dfrac{16 \text{ oz.}}{1 \cancel{\text{ lb.}}} = 88 \text{ ounces}$

7.3 Practice Volume Conversions

1. $\dfrac{6 \cancel{\text{ T.}}}{1} \cdot \dfrac{3 \text{ tsp.}}{1 \cancel{\text{ T.}}} = 18 \text{ teaspoons}$

2. $\dfrac{20 \cancel{\text{ qt.}}}{1} \cdot \dfrac{2 \text{ pt.}}{1 \cancel{\text{ qt.}}} = 40 \text{ pints}$

3. $\dfrac{4 \cancel{\text{ gal.}}}{1} \cdot \dfrac{4 \text{ qt.}}{1 \cancel{\text{ gal.}}} = 16 \text{ quarts}$

4. $\dfrac{45 \cancel{\text{ pt.}}}{1} \cdot \dfrac{2 \text{ cups}}{1 \cancel{\text{ pt.}}} = 90 \text{ cups}$

5. $\dfrac{\cancel{12}^{3} \text{ fl. oz.}}{1} \cdot \dfrac{1 \text{ cup}}{_2\cancel{8} \text{ fl. oz.}} = \dfrac{3}{2} = 1\dfrac{1}{2}$ cups

6. $\dfrac{6 \text{ gal.}}{1} \cdot \dfrac{4 \text{ qt.}}{1 \text{ gal.}} = 24$ quarts

7. $\dfrac{\cancel{27}^{9} \text{ tsp.}}{1} \cdot \dfrac{1 \text{ T.}}{_1\cancel{3} \text{ tsp.}} = 9$ tablespoons

8. $\dfrac{\cancel{10}^{5} \text{ cups}}{1} \cdot \dfrac{1 \text{ pt.}}{_1\cancel{2} \text{ cups}} = 5$ pints

9. $\dfrac{\cancel{22}^{11} \text{ qt.}}{1} \cdot \dfrac{1 \text{ gal.}}{_2\cancel{4} \text{ qt.}} = \dfrac{11}{2} = 5\dfrac{1}{2}$ gallons

10. $\dfrac{\cancel{9}^{3} \text{ tsp.}}{1} \cdot \dfrac{1 \text{ T.}}{_1\cancel{3} \text{ tsp.}} = 3$ tablespoons

11. $\dfrac{26 \text{ T.}}{1} \cdot \dfrac{}{\text{T.}} \cdot \dfrac{1 \text{ cup}}{}$

   $\dfrac{\cancel{26}^{13} \text{ T.}}{1} \cdot \dfrac{1 \text{ fl. oz.}}{_1\cancel{2} \text{ T.}} \cdot \dfrac{1 \text{ cup}}{8 \text{ fl. oz.}} = \dfrac{13}{8} = 1\dfrac{5}{8}$ cups

12. $\dfrac{2 \text{ pt.}}{1} \cdot \dfrac{}{\text{pt.}} \cdot \dfrac{\text{fl. oz.}}{}$

   $\dfrac{2 \text{ pt.}}{1} \cdot \dfrac{2 \text{ cups}}{1 \text{ pt.}} \cdot \dfrac{8 \text{ fl. oz.}}{1 \text{ cup}} = 32$ fluid ounces

13. $\dfrac{7 \text{ cups}}{1} \cdot \dfrac{}{\text{cup}} \cdot \dfrac{\text{qt.}}{}$

   $\dfrac{7 \text{ cups}}{1} \cdot \dfrac{1 \text{ pt.}}{2 \text{ cups}} \cdot \dfrac{1 \text{ qt.}}{2 \text{ pt.}} = \dfrac{7}{4} = 1\dfrac{3}{4}$ quarts

14. $\dfrac{10 \text{ gal.}}{1} \cdot \dfrac{}{\text{gal.}} \cdot \dfrac{\text{pt.}}{}$

$\dfrac{10 \cancel{\text{ gal.}}}{1} \cdot \dfrac{4 \cancel{\text{ qt.}}}{1 \cancel{\text{ gal.}}} \cdot \dfrac{2 \text{ pt.}}{1 \cancel{\text{ qt.}}} = 80 \text{ pints}$

15. $\dfrac{8 \text{ fl. oz.}}{1} \cdot \dfrac{}{\text{fl. oz.}} \cdot \dfrac{\text{pt.}}{}$

$\dfrac{\overset{1}{\cancel{8 \text{ fl. oz.}}}}{1} \cdot \dfrac{1 \text{ cup}}{\underset{1}{\cancel{8 \text{ fl. oz.}}}} \cdot \dfrac{1 \text{ pt.}}{2 \cancel{\text{ cups}}} = \dfrac{1}{2} \text{ pint}$

16. $1\dfrac{1}{2} \text{ cups} = 1.5 \text{ cups}$ $\qquad \dfrac{1.5 \text{ cups}}{1} \cdot \dfrac{}{\text{cup}} \cdot \dfrac{\text{T.}}{}$

$\dfrac{1.5 \cancel{\text{ cups}}}{1} \cdot \dfrac{8 \cancel{\text{ fl. oz.}}}{1 \cancel{\text{ cup}}} \cdot \dfrac{2 \text{ T.}}{1 \cancel{\text{ fl. oz.}}} = 24 \text{ tablespoons}$

17. $\dfrac{32 \text{ fl. oz.}}{1} \cdot \dfrac{}{\text{fl. oz.}} \cdot \dfrac{\text{pt.}}{}$

$\dfrac{\overset{2}{\underset{4}{\cancel{32 \text{ fl. oz.}}}}}{1} \cdot \dfrac{1 \text{ cup}}{\underset{1}{\cancel{8 \text{ fl. oz.}}}} \cdot \dfrac{1 \text{ pt.}}{\underset{1}{\cancel{2 \text{ cups}}}} = 2 \text{ pints}$

18. $\dfrac{160 \text{ cups}}{1} \cdot \dfrac{}{\text{cup}} \cdot \dfrac{\text{qt.}}{}$

$\dfrac{\overset{40}{\underset{80}{\cancel{160 \text{ cups}}}}}{1} \cdot \dfrac{1 \text{ pt.}}{\underset{1}{\cancel{2 \text{ cups}}}} \cdot \dfrac{1 \text{ qt.}}{\underset{1}{\cancel{2 \text{ pt.}}}} = 40 \text{ quarts}$

19. $\dfrac{32 \text{ T.}}{1} \cdot \dfrac{}{\text{T.}} \cdot \dfrac{\text{cups}}{}$

$\dfrac{\overset{2}{\underset{16}{\cancel{32 \text{ T.}}}}}{1} \cdot \dfrac{1 \text{ fl. oz.}}{\underset{1}{\cancel{2 \text{ T.}}}} \cdot \dfrac{1 \text{ cup}}{\underset{1}{\cancel{8 \text{ fl. oz.}}}} = 2 \text{ cups}$

20. $\dfrac{3 \text{ qt.}}{1} \cdot \dfrac{}{\text{qt.}} \cdot \dfrac{\text{cups}}{}$

$\dfrac{3 \cancel{\text{ qt.}}}{1} \cdot \dfrac{2 \cancel{\text{ pt.}}}{1 \cancel{\text{ qt.}}} \cdot \dfrac{2 \text{ cups}}{1 \cancel{\text{ pt.}}} = 12 \text{ cups}$

7.4 Chapter Test for Household Measures

Sections 7.1, 7.2, and 7.3

1. $\dfrac{5 \ \cancel{T.}}{1} \bullet \dfrac{3 \ tsp.}{1 \ \cancel{T.}} = 15 \ teaspoons$

2. $\dfrac{\overset{5}{\cancel{20}} \ in.}{1} \bullet \dfrac{1 \ ft.}{\underset{3}{\cancel{12}} \ in.} = \dfrac{5}{3} = 1\dfrac{2}{3} \ feet$

3. $7\dfrac{1}{2} \ pints = 7.5 \ pints$

   $\dfrac{7.5 \ \cancel{pt.}}{1} \bullet \dfrac{2 \ cups}{1 \ \cancel{pt.}} = 15 \ cups$

4. $\dfrac{7 \ \cancel{T.}}{1} \bullet \dfrac{1 \ fl. \ oz.}{2 \ \cancel{T.}} = \dfrac{7}{2} = 3\dfrac{1}{2} \ fluid \ ounces$

5. $\dfrac{\overset{6}{\cancel{18}} \ tsp.}{1} \bullet \dfrac{1 \ T.}{\underset{1}{\cancel{3}} \ tsp.} = 6 \ tablespoons$

6. $\dfrac{9 \ \cancel{pt.}}{1} \bullet \dfrac{1 \ qt.}{2 \ \cancel{pt.}} = \dfrac{9}{2} = 4\dfrac{1}{2} \ quarts$

7. $\dfrac{3.5 \ \cancel{tons}}{1} \bullet \dfrac{2,000 \ lb.}{1 \ \cancel{ton}} = 7,000 \ pounds$

8. $\dfrac{4.6 \ \cancel{mi.}}{1} \bullet \dfrac{5,280 \ ft.}{1 \ \cancel{mi.}} = 24,288 \ feet$

9. $\dfrac{\overset{7}{\cancel{14}} \ fl. \ oz.}{1} \bullet \dfrac{1 \ cup}{\underset{4}{\cancel{8}} \ fl. \ oz.} = \dfrac{7}{4} = 1\dfrac{3}{4} \ cups$

10. $\dfrac{\overset{\overset{1}{264}}{\cancel{2,640}} \ ft.}{1} \bullet \dfrac{1 \ mi.}{\underset{2}{\underset{528}{\cancel{5,280}}} \ ft.} = \dfrac{1}{2} \ mile$

11. $\dfrac{3 \text{ fl. oz.}}{1} \cdot \dfrac{2 \text{ T.}}{1 \text{ fl. oz.}}$ = 6 tablespoons

12. $\dfrac{\overset{3}{\cancel{6} \text{ qt.}}}{1} \cdot \dfrac{1 \text{ gal.}}{\underset{2}{\cancel{4} \text{ qt.}}} = \dfrac{3}{2} = 1\dfrac{1}{2}$ gallons

13. $\dfrac{1.5 \text{ lb.}}{1} \cdot \dfrac{16 \text{ oz.}}{1 \text{ lb.}}$ = 24 ounces

14. $\dfrac{\overset{27}{\cancel{81} \text{ ft.}}}{1} \cdot \dfrac{1 \text{ yd.}}{\underset{1}{\cancel{3} \text{ ft.}}}$ = 27 yards

15. $\dfrac{\overset{1}{\cancel{4} \text{ fl. oz.}}}{1} \cdot \dfrac{1 \text{ cup}}{\underset{2}{\cancel{8} \text{ fl. oz.}}} = \dfrac{1}{2}$ cup

16. $\dfrac{12 \text{ qt.}}{1} \cdot \dfrac{2 \text{ pt.}}{1 \text{ qt.}}$ = 24 pints

17. $3\dfrac{1}{2}$ feet = 3.5 feet

$\dfrac{3.5 \text{ ft.}}{1} \cdot \dfrac{12 \text{ in.}}{1 \text{ ft.}}$ = 42 inches

Section 7.3

18. $\dfrac{4 \text{ pt.}}{1} \cdot \dfrac{}{\text{pt.}} \cdot \dfrac{\text{fl. oz.}}{}$

$\dfrac{4 \text{ pt.}}{1} \cdot \dfrac{2 \text{ cups}}{1 \text{ pt.}} \cdot \dfrac{8 \text{ fl. oz.}}{1 \text{ cup}}$ = 64 fluid ounces

19. $\dfrac{2 \text{ cups}}{1} \cdot \dfrac{}{\text{cup}} \cdot \dfrac{\text{qt.}}{}$

$\dfrac{\overset{1}{\cancel{2} \text{ cups}}}{1} \cdot \dfrac{1 \text{ pt.}}{\underset{1}{\cancel{2} \text{ cups}}} \cdot \dfrac{1 \text{ qt.}}{2 \text{ pt.}} = \dfrac{1}{2} \text{ quart}$

20. $\dfrac{2.5 \text{ fl. oz.}}{1} \cdot \dfrac{}{\text{fl. oz.}} \cdot \dfrac{\text{tsp.}}{}$

$\dfrac{2.5 \text{ fl. oz.}}{1} \cdot \dfrac{2 \text{ T.}}{1 \text{ fl. oz.}} \cdot \dfrac{3 \text{ tsp.}}{1 \text{ T.}} = 15 \text{ teaspoons}$

8.0　　　**Pretest for the Metric System**

Section 8.1

1. 52.467 • 100 **= 52.46.7 = 5,246.7**

2. 897.2 ÷ 10,000 **= .0897.2 = 0.08972**

Section 8.2

3. 1 kg = **1,000** g

4. 1 mm = **0.001** m

5. 1 g = **1,000,000** mcg

Sections 8.3 and 8.4

6. 75,000 g = **75** kg　　　**75.000 = 75**

7. 5 m = **500** cm　　　**5.00. = 500**

8. 1.4 m = **1,400** mm　　　**1.400. = 1,400**

9. 34.5 mg = **0.0345** g　　　**.034.5 = 0.0345**

10. 5.3 mL = **0.0053** L　　　**.005.3 = 0.0053**

8.1 Practice Multiplication and Division by Powers of 10

1. 3.46 • 100 **= 3.46. = 346**

2. 45.61 ÷ 1,000 **= .045.61 = 0.04561**

3. 78.4 ÷ 100 **= .78.4 = 0.784**

4. 0.435 • 10 = **0.4.35 = 4.35**

5. 1.54 ÷ 10,000 = **.0001.54 = 0.000154**

6. 4.1782 • 1,000 = **4.178.2 = 4,178.2**

7. 167 ÷ 10 = **16.7. = 16.7**

8. 16.493 ÷ 100 = **.16.493 = 0.16493**

9. 0.00615 • 10,000 = **0.0061.5 = 61.5**

10. 1.86 • 10 = **1.8.6 = 18.6**

11. 20.57 • 100 = **20.57. = 2,057**

12. 73.85 ÷ 1,000 = **.073.85 = 0.07385**

13. 0.38 • 1,000 = **0.380. = 380**

14. 157.1 ÷ 10 = **15.7.1 = 15.71**

15. 169.9 ÷ 10,000 = **.0169.9 = 0.01699**

16. 0.719 • 10 = **0.7.19 = 7.19**

17. 24.5 ÷ 1,000 = **.024.5 = 0.0245**

18. 7.4 • 10,000 = **7.4000. = 74,000**

19. 38.2 • 100 = **38.20. = 3,820**

20. 10.413 ÷ 10,000 = **.0010.413 = 0.0010413**

8.2 Practice Metric System Basics

1. deca = **da**

2. milli = **m**

3. centi = **c**

4. kilo = **k**

5. micro = **mc**

6. centi = **0.01 or** $\dfrac{1}{100}$

7. kilo = **1,000**

8. micro = **0.000001 or** $\dfrac{1}{1,000,000}$

9. milli = **0.001 or** $\dfrac{1}{1,000}$

10. (g) or mg
    g = 1g   mg = 0.001g
    1g > 0.001g
    Gram is larger.

11. g or (kg)
    g = 1g   kg = 1,000g
    1g < 1,000g
    Kilogram is larger.

12. mcg or (g)
    1mcg = 0.000001g   g = 1g
    0.000001g < 1g
    Gram is larger.

13. (m) or mm
    m = 1m   1mm = 0.001m
    1m > 0.001m
    Meter is larger.

14. ⓚ or m

  1km = 1,000m   m = 1m
      1,000 m > 1m
      Kilometer is larger.

15. mL or Ⓛ

  1mL = 0.001L   L = 1L
      0.001L < 1L
      Liter is larger.

16. ⓜ or cm

  m = 1m   1cm = 0.01m
      1m > 0.01m
      Meter is larger.

17. 10^3 = 1,000

18. 10^{-6} = 0.000001 or $\dfrac{1}{1,000,000}$

19. 10^{-3} = 0.001 or $\dfrac{1}{1,000}$

20. 10^6 = 1,000,000

8.3 Practice Metric Units Used in Nursing

1. 1 meter is a little longer than a yardstick.

2. 1 centimeter is the approximate diameter of a dime.

3. 1 gram is the weight of a paper clip.

4. 1 milligram is the weight of a pinch of salt.

5. 1 millimeter is the approximate thickness of a CD.

6. 1 kilogram is the weight of slightly more than a quart of water.

7. 1 milliliter is approximately one drip from a faucet.

8. 1g = <u>**1,000**</u> mg

9. 1,000 g = <u>**1**</u> kg

10. 0.000001g = <u>**1**</u> mcg

11. 1mg = <u>**1,000**</u> mcg

12. 1km = <u>**1,000**</u> m

13. 1,000,000 mcg = <u>**1**</u> g

14. 1m = <u>**100**</u> cm

15. 1,000 mL = <u>**1**</u> L

16. 1mg = <u>**0.001**</u> g

17. 1m = <u>**0.001**</u> km

18. 1mm = <u>**0.1**</u> cm

19. 1,000 mm = <u>**1**</u> m

20. 1cm = <u>**0.01**</u> m

8.4 Practice Converting Units in the Metric System

1. 12 m = **1,200** cm   Meters are larger than centimeters, so multiply.

    1m = 100 cm

      100 = 10^2

   12.00. = 1,200

2. 34.6 g = **34,600** mg   Grams are larger than milligrams, so multiply.

    1g = 1,000 mg

    1,000 = 10^3

  34.600. = 34,600

3. 48 mm = <u>0.048</u> m   Millimeters are smaller than meters, so divide.
    1,000 mm = 1 m
        1,000 = 10^3
        .048. = 0.048
        ⌣⌣⌣

4. 75 mcg = <u>0.075</u> mg   Micrograms are smaller than milligrams, so
    1,000 mcg = 1 mg   divide.
        1,000 = 10^3
        .075. = 0.075
        ⌣⌣⌣

5. 735 mg = <u>0.735</u> g   Milligrams are smaller than grams, so divide.
    1,000 mg = 1 g
        1,000 = 10^3
        .735. = 0.735
        ⌣⌣⌣

6. 2 mL = <u>0.002</u> L   Milliliters are smaller than liters, so divide.
    1,000 mL = 1 L
        1,000 = 10^3
        .002. = 0.002
        ⌣⌣⌣

7. 0.3 m = <u>300</u> mm   Meters are larger than millimeters, so multiply.
        1 m = 1,000 mm
        1,000 = 10^3
      0.300. = 300
        ⌣⌣⌣

8.   73 kg = <u>73,000,000</u> mg   Kilograms are larger than milligrams,
        1 kg = 1,000,000 mg   so multiply.
        1,000,000 = 10^6
      73.000000. = 73,000,000
        ⌣⌣⌣⌣⌣⌣

9. 3.4 L = <u>3,400</u> mL   Liters are larger than milliliters, so multiply.
        1 L = 1,000 mL
        1,000 = 10^3
      3.400. = 3,400
        ⌣⌣⌣

10. 6.4 cm = <u>0.064</u> m   Centimeters are smaller than meters, so divide.
    100 cm = 1 m
       100 = 10^2
    .06.4 = 0.064
     ⌣⌣

11. 7,480 g = <u>7.48</u> kg   Grams are smaller than kilograms, so divide.
     1 g = 1,000 kg
   1,000 = 10^3
  7.480. = 7.480̸ = 7.48
   ⌣⌣⌣

12. 536 cm³ = <u>536</u> mL   Cubic centimeters and milliliters are equal.
    1 cm³ = 1 mL

13.   2 mcg = <u>0.002</u> mg   Micrograms are smaller than milligrams, so
  1,000 mcg = 1 mg   divide.
    1,000 = 10^3
    .002. = 0.002
   ⌣⌣⌣

14. 528 cm = <u>5.28</u> m   Centimeters are smaller than meters, so divide.
   100 cm = 1 m
    100 = 10^2
   5.28. = 5.28
   ⌣⌣

15.   50 L = <u>50,000</u> mL   Liters are larger than milliliters, so multiply.
    1 L = 1,000 mL
   1,000 = 10^3
  50.000. = 50,000
    ⌣⌣⌣

16. 0.54 g = <u>540</u> mg   Grams are larger than milligrams, so multiply.
    1 g = 1,000 mg
   1,000 = 10^3
  0.540. = 540
   ⌣⌣⌣

17.   12 mg = <u>12,000</u> mcg   Milligrams are larger than micrograms, so
    1 mg = 1,000 mcg   multiply.
   1,000 = 10^3
  12.000. = 12,000
   ⌣⌣⌣

18. 2.27 mL = <u>0.00227</u> L   Milliliters are smaller than liters, so divide.

1,000 mL = 1 L

1,000 = 10^3

.002.27 = 0.00227

19. 25 mm = <u>2.5</u> cm   Millimeters are smaller than centimeters, so divide.

10 mm = 1 cm

10 = 10^1

2.5. = 2.5

20.   896 g = <u>896,000</u> mg   Grams are larger than milligrams, so multiply.

1 g = 1,000 mg

1,000 = 10^3

896.000. = 896,000

8.5 Chapter Test for the Metric System

Section 8.1

1. 27.45 • 1,000 = 27.450. = 27,450

2. 0.23 ÷ 10 = .0.23 = 0.023

3. 15.642 • 100 = 15.64.2 = 1,564.2

4. 9.1 ÷ 10,000 = .0009.1 = 0.00091

Section 8.2

5. kilo has a value of <u>1,000</u>

6. centi has a value of <u>0.01</u>

7. milli has a value of <u>0.001</u>

8. micro has a value of <u>0.000001</u>

Sections 8.3 and 8.4

9. $1\,cm^3 = \underline{\ 1\ }\,mL$ Cubic centimeters and milliliters are equal.

10. $275\,mcg = \underline{0.275}\,mg$ Micrograms are smaller than milligrams,
   $1,000\,mcg = 1\,mg$ so divide.
       $1,000 = 10^3$
       $.275. = 0.275$
       ⌣⌣⌣

11. $135\,mg = \underline{0.135}\,g$ Milligrams are smaller than grams, so divide.
   $1,000\,mg = 1\,g$
       $1,000 = 10^3$
       $.135. = 0.135$
       ⌣⌣⌣

12. $3.1\,cm = \underline{31}\,mm$ Centimeters are larger than millimeters,
       $1\,cm = 10\,mm$ so multiply.
        $10 = 10^1$
        $3.1. = 31$
           ⌣

13. $2\,mg = \underline{2,000}\,mcg$ Milligrams are larger than micrograms,
       $1\,mg = 1,000\,mcg$ so multiply.
     $1,000 = 10^3$
     $2.000. = 2,000$
        ⌣⌣⌣

14. $2.5\,kg = \underline{2,500}\,g$ Kilograms are larger than grams, so multiply.
       $1\,kg = 1,000\,g$
     $1,000 = 10^3$
     $2.500. = 2,500$
        ⌣⌣⌣

15. $569\,mL = \underline{0.569}\,L$ Milliliters are smaller than liters, so divide.
   $1,000\,mL = 1\,L$
       $1,000 = 10^3$
       $.569. = 0.569$
       ⌣⌣⌣

16. 0.8 mcg = <u>0.0008</u> mg   Micrograms are smaller than milligrams,
    1,000 mcg = 1 mg   so divide.
        $1,000 = 10^3$
        .000.8 = 0.0008
        ⌣⌣⌣

17. 6.37 mL = <u>0.00637</u> L Milliliters are smaller than liters, so divide.
    1,000 mL = 1 L
        $1,000 = 10^3$
        .006.37 = 0.00637
        ⌣⌣⌣

18. 5,600 g = <u>5.6</u> kg   Grams are smaller than kilograms, so divide.
    1,000 g = 1 kg
        $1,000 = 10^3$
    5.600. = 5.6~~00~~ = 5.6
        ⌣⌣⌣

19. 3.2 L = <u>3,200</u> mL   Liters are larger than milliliters, so multiply.
        1 L = 1,000 mL
    $1,000 = 10^3$
    3.200. = 3,200
        ⌣⌣⌣

20.   0.3 g = <u>300,000</u> mcg   Grams are larger than micrograms, so
        1 g = 1,000,000 mcg   multiply.
    $1,000,000 = 10^6$
    0.300000. = 300,000
        ⌣⌣⌣⌣⌣⌣

Practice Test 1
Basic Unit Conversions for Household and Metric Measures

Section

(8.3) 1. 1 m = **100** cm

(7.2) 2. 1 ton = **2,000** lb.

(7.3) 3. 1 cup = **8** fl. oz.

(8.3) 4. 1 kg = **1,000** g

(7.1) 5. 12 in. = **1** ft.

(7.3) 6. 1 T. = **3** tsp.

(8.3) 7. 1,000 mm = **1** m

(7.1) 8. 1 mi. = **5,280** ft.

(8.3) 9. 10 mm = **1** cm

(7.3) 10. 2 pt. = **1** qt.

(7.3) 11. 2 T. = **1** fl. oz.

(8.3) 12. 0.001 g = **1** mg

(7.1) 13. 1 yd. = **3** ft.

(7.2) 14. 1 lb. = **16** oz.

(8.3) 15. 1,000,000 mcg = **1** g

(7.3) 16. 1 gal. = **4** qt.

(8.3) 17. $27 \, cm^3$ = **27** mL

(8.3) 18. 1 L = **1,000** mL

(7.3) 19. 1 pt. = **2** cups

(8.3) 20. 1 mcg = **0.000001** g

SOLUTIONS

Practice Test 2
Performing Household
and Metric Conversions

Section

(7.1) 1. $\dfrac{\overset{7}{\cancel{84}} \text{ in.}}{1} \cdot \dfrac{1\,\text{ft.}}{\underset{1}{\cancel{12}}\text{ in.}} = 7 \text{ feet}$

(7.3) 2. $\dfrac{31\,\cancel{\text{pt.}}}{1} \cdot \dfrac{2\,\text{cups}}{1\,\cancel{\text{pt.}}} = 62 \text{ cups}$

(7.3) 3. $\dfrac{2\,\cancel{\text{gal.}}}{1} \cdot \dfrac{4\,\cancel{\text{qt.}}}{1\,\cancel{\text{gal.}}} \cdot \dfrac{2\,\text{pt.}}{1\,\cancel{\text{qt.}}} = 16 \text{ pints}$

(7.1) 4. $\dfrac{41\,\cancel{\text{yd.}}}{1} \cdot \dfrac{3\,\text{ft.}}{1\,\cancel{\text{yd.}}} = 123 \text{ feet}$

(7.3) 5. $\dfrac{\overset{3}{\cancel{12}}\,\cancel{\text{T.}}}{1} \cdot \dfrac{1\,\cancel{\text{fl. oz.}}}{2\,\cancel{\text{T.}}} \cdot \dfrac{1\,\text{cup}}{\underset{2}{\cancel{8}}\,\cancel{\text{fl. oz.}}} = \dfrac{3}{4} \text{ cup}$

(7.3) 6. $\dfrac{3\,\cancel{\text{cups}}}{1} \cdot \dfrac{8\,\text{fl. oz.}}{1\,\cancel{\text{cup}}} = 24 \text{ fluid ounces}$

(7.1) 7. $\dfrac{\overset{2}{\cancel{10{,}560}}\,\cancel{\text{ft.}}}{1} \cdot \dfrac{1\,\text{mi.}}{\underset{1}{\cancel{5{,}280}}\,\cancel{\text{ft.}}} = 2 \text{ miles}$

(7.3) 8. $\dfrac{8\,\cancel{\text{fl. oz.}}}{1} \cdot \dfrac{2\,\text{T.}}{1\,\cancel{\text{fl. oz.}}} = 16 \text{ tablespoons}$

(7.3) 9. $2\dfrac{1}{2} \text{ qt.} = 2.5\,\text{qt.} \quad \dfrac{2.5\,\cancel{\text{qt.}}}{1} \cdot \dfrac{4\,\text{cups}}{1\,\cancel{\text{qt.}}} = 10 \text{ cups}$

(7.3) 10. $\dfrac{6\,\cancel{\text{gal.}}}{1} \cdot \dfrac{4\,\text{qt.}}{1\,\cancel{\text{gal.}}} = 24 \text{ quarts}$

(7.3) 11. $\dfrac{2 \text{ q̶t̶.}}{1} \cdot \dfrac{2\,\text{pt.}}{1\,\text{q̶t̶.}} = 4\ \text{pints}$

(7.1) 12. $\dfrac{17\ \text{f̶t̶.}}{1} \cdot \dfrac{12\,\text{in.}}{1\,\text{f̶t̶.}} = 204\ \text{inches}$

(7.3) 13. $\dfrac{\overset{7}{\cancel{14\ \text{fl. oz.}}}}{1} \cdot \dfrac{1\ \text{cup}}{\underset{4}{\cancel{8\ \text{fl. oz.}}}} \cdot \dfrac{1\,\text{pt.}}{2\,\text{cups}} = \dfrac{7}{8}\ \text{pint}$

(7.3) 14. $\dfrac{\overset{3}{\cancel{9\ \text{tsp.}}}}{1} \cdot \dfrac{1\,\text{T.}}{\underset{1}{\cancel{3\ \text{tsp.}}}} = 3\ \text{tablespoons}$

(7.3) 15. $\dfrac{2\ \text{p̶t̶.}}{1} \cdot \dfrac{2\,\text{cups}}{1\,\text{p̶t̶.}} \cdot \dfrac{8\,\text{fl. oz.}}{1\,\text{cup}} = 32\ \text{fluid ounces}$

(7.2) 16. $\dfrac{13\ \text{tons}}{1} \cdot \dfrac{2{,}000\,\text{lb.}}{1\,\text{ton}} = 26{,}000\ \text{pounds}$

(7.3) 17. $\dfrac{\overset{5}{\cancel{10\ \text{T.}}}}{1} \cdot \dfrac{1\,\text{fl. oz.}}{\underset{1}{\cancel{2\ \text{T.}}}} = 5\ \text{fluid ounces}$

(7.1) 18. $\dfrac{\overset{4}{\cancel{12\ \text{ft.}}}}{1} \cdot \dfrac{1\,\text{yd.}}{\underset{1}{\cancel{3\ \text{ft.}}}} = 4\ \text{yards}$

(7.3) 19. $\dfrac{\overset{1}{\cancel{8\ \text{fl. oz.}}}}{1} \cdot \dfrac{1\,\text{cup}}{\underset{1}{\cancel{8\ \text{fl. oz.}}}} \cdot \dfrac{1\,\text{pt.}}{2\,\text{cups}} = \dfrac{1}{2}\ \text{pint}$

(7.2) 20. $\dfrac{4\ \text{l̶b̶.}}{1} \cdot \dfrac{16\,\text{oz.}}{1\,\text{l̶b̶.}} = 64\ \text{ounces}$

(7.3) 21. $\dfrac{\overset{9}{\cancel{18\ \text{pt.}}}}{1} \cdot \dfrac{1\,\text{qt.}}{\underset{1}{\cancel{2\ \text{pt.}}}} = 9\ \text{quarts}$

(7.3) 22. $\dfrac{2\ \text{cups}}{1} \cdot \dfrac{8\,\text{fl. oz.}}{1\,\text{cup}} = 16\ \text{fluid ounces}$

(7.2) 23. $\dfrac{\overset{9}{\cancel{144}}\ \cancel{oz.}}{1} \cdot \dfrac{1\ lb.}{\underset{1}{\cancel{16}}\ \cancel{oz.}} = 9\ pounds$

(7.3) 24. $\dfrac{\overset{4}{\cancel{32}}\ \cancel{fl.\ oz.}}{1} \cdot \dfrac{1\ cup}{\underset{1}{\cancel{8\ fl.\ oz.}}} = 4\ cups$

(7.1) 25. $\dfrac{\overset{6}{\cancel{31,680}}\ \cancel{ft.}}{1} \cdot \dfrac{1\ mi.}{\underset{1}{\cancel{5,280}}\ \cancel{ft.}} = 6\ miles$

(7.3) 26. $\dfrac{\overset{27}{\cancel{54}}\ \cancel{cups}}{1} \cdot \dfrac{1\ pt.}{\underset{1}{\cancel{2}}\ \cancel{cups}} = 27\ pints$

(7.3) 27. $\dfrac{7}{8}\ pt. = 0.875\ pt.$ $\dfrac{0.875\ \cancel{pt.}}{1} \cdot \dfrac{2\ \cancel{cups}}{1\ \cancel{pt.}} \cdot \dfrac{8\ fl.\ oz.}{1\ \cancel{cup}} = 14\ fluid\ ounces$

(7.1) 28. $\dfrac{\overset{15}{\cancel{180}}\ \cancel{in.}}{1} \cdot \dfrac{1\ ft.}{\underset{1}{\cancel{12}}\ \cancel{in.}} = 15\ feet$

(7.3) 29. $\dfrac{\overset{7}{\cancel{28}}\ \cancel{qt.}}{1} \cdot \dfrac{1\ gal.}{\underset{1}{\cancel{4}}\ \cancel{qt.}} = 7\ gallons$

(7.3) 30. $\dfrac{6\ \cancel{T.}}{1} \cdot \dfrac{3\ tsp.}{1\ \cancel{T.}} = 18\ teaspoons$

(7.3) 31. $\dfrac{2\ \cancel{fl.\ oz.}}{1} \cdot \dfrac{2\ T.}{1\ \cancel{fl.\ oz.}} = 4\ tablespoons$

(7.3) 32. $\dfrac{4\ \cancel{qt.}}{1} \cdot \dfrac{2\ \cancel{pt.}}{1\ \cancel{qt.}} \cdot \dfrac{2\ cups}{1\ \cancel{pt.}} = 16\ cups$

(7.2) 33. $\dfrac{\overset{17}{\cancel{34,000}}\ \cancel{lb.}}{1} \cdot \dfrac{1\ ton}{\underset{1}{\cancel{2,000}}\ \cancel{lb.}} = 17\ tons$

(8.4) 34. 46.8 m = <u>4,680</u> cm

1 m = 100 cm

$100 = 10^2$

4 6.8 0. = 4,680

Meters are larger than centimeters, so multiply.

(8.4) 35. 3.162 kg = <u>3,162</u> g

1 kg = 1,000 g

$1,000 = 10^3$

3.1 6 2. = 3,162

Kilograms are larger than grams, so multiply.

(8.4) 36. 27 mm = <u>0.027</u> m

1,000 mm = 1 m

$1,000 = 10^3$

.0 2 7. = 0.027

Millimeters are smaller than meters, so divide.

(8.4) 37. 426 mcg = <u>0.426</u> mg

1,000 mcg = 1 mg

$1,000 = 10^3$

.4 2 6. = 0.426

Micrograms are smaller than milligrams, so divide.

(8.4) 38. 3.82 L = <u>3,820</u> mL

1 L = 1,000 mL

$1,000 = 10^3$

3.8 2 0. = 3,820

Liters are larger than milliliters, so multiply.

(8.4) 39. 98.6 cm = <u>986</u> mm

1 cm = 10 mm

$10 = 10^1$

9 8.6. = 986

Centimeters are larger than millimeters, so multiply.

(8.4) 40. 75 mL = <u>75</u> cm^3

1 mL = 1 cm^3

Milliliters and cubic centimeters are equal.

(8.4) 41. 0.568 g = <u>568</u> mg

1 g = 1,000 mg

$1,000 = 10^3$

0.5 6 8. = 568

Grams are larger than milligrams, so multiply.

(8.4) 42. 0.014 g = <u>14,000</u> mcg   Grams are larger than micrograms,
           1 g = 1,000,000 mcg   so multiply.

$$1,000,000 = 10^6$$
$$0.014000. = 14,000$$

(8.4) 43. 5,300 mL = <u>5.3</u> L   Milliliters are smaller than liters, so
     1,000 mL = 1 L   divide.

$$1,000 = 10^3$$
$$5.300. = 5.300 = 5.3$$

(8.4) 44. 5,296 mm = <u>529.6</u> cm   Millimeters are smaller than
      10 mm = 1 cm   centimeters, so divide.

$$10 = 10^1$$
$$529.6. = 529.6$$

(8.4) 45. 13 mg = <u>0.013</u> g   Milligrams are smaller than grams, so
    1,000 mg = 1 g   divide.

$$1,000 = 10^3$$
$$.013. = 0.013$$

(8.4) 46. 294 g = <u>0.294</u> kg   Grams are smaller than kilograms, so
    1,000 g = 1 kg   divide.

$$1,000 = 10^3$$
$$.294. = 0.294$$

(8.4) 47. 42.8 cm = <u>0.428</u> m   Centimeters are smaller than meters, so
    100 cm = 1 m   divide.

$$100 = 10^2$$
$$0.42.8 = 0.428$$

(8.4) 48. 0.328 m = <u>328</u> mm   Meters are larger than millimeters, so
     1 m = 1,000 mm   multiply.

$$1,000 = 10^3$$
$$0.328. = 328$$

(8.4) 49.   10 mcg = <u>0.00001</u> g   Micrograms are smaller than grams,
        1,000,000 mcg = 1 g   so divide.
            1,000,000 = 10^6
            .000010. = 0.00001
            ⌣⌣⌣⌣⌣

(8.4) 50. 5 cm^3 = <u>5</u> mL   Cubic centimeters and milliliters are
                            equal.
        1 cm^3 = 1 mL

(8.4) 51. 0.25 mg = <u>250</u> mcg   Milligrams are larger than micrograms,
        1 mg = 1,000 mcg   so multiply.
        1,000 = 10^3
        0.250. = 250
            ⌣⌣⌣

(8.4) 52.   0.0975 mcg = <u>0.0000975</u> mg   Micrograms are smaller than
        1,000 mcg = 1 mg   milligrams, so divide.
            1,000 = 10^3
        0.000.0975 = 0.0000975
            ⌣⌣⌣

(8.4) 53. 0.825 m = <u>82.5</u> cm   Meters are larger than centimeters, so
        1 m = 100 cm   multiply.
        100 = 10^2
        0.82.5 = 82.5
            ⌣⌣

(8.4) 54. 45 cm^3 = <u>45</u> mL   Cubic centimeters and milliliters are
                            equal.
        1 cm^3 = 1 mL

(8.4) 55.   2 g = <u>2,000,000</u> mcg   Grams are larger than
        1 g = 1,000,000 mcg   micrograms, so multiply.
        1,000,000 = 10^6
        2.000000. = 2,000,000
            ⌣⌣⌣⌣⌣⌣

(8.4) 56.   27 mg = <u>0.027</u> g   Milligrams are smaller than grams, so
        1,000 mg = 1 g   divide.
        1,000 = 10^3
        .027. = 0.027
            ⌣⌣⌣

(8.4) 57. 37 cm = <u>370</u> mm   Centimeters are larger than millimeters,
         1 cm = 10 mm   so multiply.

          $10 = 10^1$

       37.0. = 370

(8.4) 58.   493 L = <u>493,000</u> mL   Liters are larger than milliliters, so
         1 L = 1,000 mL   multiply.

       $1,000 = 10^3$

   493.000. = 493,000

(8.4) 59. 2.92 kg = <u>2,920</u> g   Kilograms are larger than grams, so
         1 kg = 1,000 g   multiply.

       $1,000 = 10^3$

    2.920. = 2,920

(8.4) 60. 508 mm = <u>0.508</u> m   Millimeters are smaller than meters, so
     1,000 mm = 1 m   divide.

       $1,000 = 10^3$

     .508. = 0.508

Roman Numerals

In this appendix, we will review:
- seven basic symbols
- reading and writing Roman numerals

Seven Basic Symbols

Nursing students must be able to interpret Roman numerals. Occasionally, doctors use Roman numerals for indicating the quantity of a medication on their written orders or prescriptions.

The Roman system uses seven symbols to represent whole numbers.

I, i = 1
V, v = 5
X, x = 10
L, l = 50
C, c = 100
D, d = 500
M, m = 1,000

In nursing, i for 1, v for 5, and x for 10 are the most commonly used numerals. The lowercase (i, v, x) is used more often than the uppercase (I, V, X).

Reading and Writing Roman Numerals

Using definite rules, the seven basic numerals can be combined to represent other numbers. These same rules apply to both reading and writing Roman numerals.

Rule 1: When a smaller numeral follows a larger numeral, add the two numerals. For example:

vi = 6	5 + 1 = 6
xv = 15	10 + 5 = 15
xvi = 16	10 + 5 + 1 = 16

Rule 2: When a numeral is repeated, add the numerals. However, a numeral is never repeated more than three times. For example:

ii = 2	$1 + 1 = 2$
viii = 8	$5 + 1 + 1 + 1 = 8$
xxiii = 23	$10 + 10 + 1 + 1 + 1 = 23$

Tip: These three Roman numerals are never written twice because the resulting value would equal one of the basic symbols:
x = 10, do not use vv $(5 + 5 = 10)$
c = 100, do not use ll $(50 + 50 = 100)$
m = 1,000, do not use dd $(500 + 500 = 1,000)$

Rule 3: When a smaller numeral is in front of a larger one, subtract. Remember, a numeral cannot be repeated more than three times; therefore, subtraction is used to represent 4s and 9s. For example:

iv = 4	$5 - 1 = 4$
ix = 9	$10 - 1 = 9$
xc = 90	$100 - 10 = 90$

Rule 4: When a smaller numeral is between two larger numerals, subtract the smaller numeral from the larger numeral to the right. For example:

xiv = 14	$10 + (5 - 1) = 10 + 4 = 14$
xxix = 29	$(10 + 10) + (10 - 1) = 20 + 9 = 29$
xliv = 44	$(50 - 10) + (5 - 1) = 40 + 4 = 44$

Temperature Conversions

In this appendix, we will review:
- Fahrenheit and Celsius temperatures
- the basis for the conversion formulas
- temperature conversion formulas

Fahrenheit and Celsius Temperatures

Two measures are predominantly used for reading temperature: **Fahrenheit** (F) is used in the United States and **Celsius** (C) is used in most other countries. Celsius also may be referred to as **Centigrade.** As the prefix **centi** indicates, this measure is part of the metric system.

These three thermometers show benchmark temperatures that are equal in the two scales.

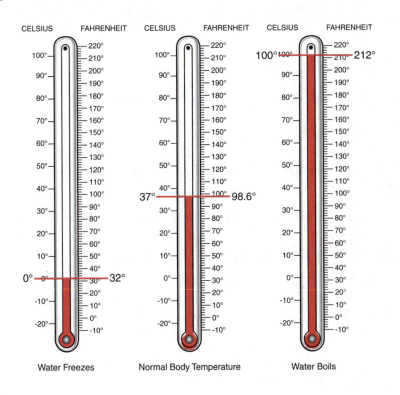

Water Freezes   Normal Body Temperature   Water Boils

The freezing temperature for water is 32°F and 0°C.
The boiling temperature for water is 212°F and 100°C.
Normal body temperature is about 98.6°F and 37°C.

Fahrenheit temperatures are always larger numbers than Celsius temperatures.

The Basis for the Conversion Formulas

The conversion formulas for Fahrenheit and Celsius are based on these considerations:

- If you compare the two scales at the freezing points 32°F and 0°C, the difference between the two is 32.
- If you compare the two scales at the boiling points, the Fahrenheit scale rises 180° from freezing to boiling (212° − 32° = 180°), and the Celsius scales rises 100° from freezing to boiling (100° − 0° = 100°). The scales are rising at a different rate, which is shown by these ratios:

$$\frac{\text{Change in Fahrenheit}}{\text{Change in Celsius}} = \frac{180}{100} = \frac{9}{5} \qquad \frac{\text{Change in Celsius}}{\text{Change in Fahrenheit}} = \frac{100}{180} = \frac{5}{9}$$

Conversion Formulas

To convert from Fahrenheit to Celsius, use this formula:

$$C = \frac{5}{9}(F - 32)$$

These are the steps for converting from Fahrenheit temperature to Celsius:

1. Substitute the Fahrenheit temperature for the letter F in the formula.
2. Subtract 32 from the Fahrenheit temperature.
3. Multiply the difference by $\frac{5}{9}$.

Example 1: Convert 86° Fahrenheit to Celsius.

STEP 1. Substitute 86 for the letter F in the formula

$C = \dfrac{5}{9} (F - 32)$.

$$C = \dfrac{5}{9} (F - 32)$$

$$C = \dfrac{5}{9} (86 - 32)$$

STEP 2. Perform the operation in parenthesis first.
Subtract: 86 − 32 = 54.

$$C = \dfrac{5}{9} (54)$$

STEP 3. Write both terms in fraction form, cross cancel, multiply, and reduce the answer.

$$C = \dfrac{5}{\cancel{9}^{1}} \cdot \dfrac{\cancel{54}^{6}}{1}$$

The answer is 86°F = 30°C.

$$C = 30$$

To convert from Celsius to Fahrenheit, use this formula:

$$F = \dfrac{9}{5} C + 32$$

These are the steps for converting from Celsius to Fahrenheit.

1. Substitute the Celsius temperature for the letter C in the formula.

2. Multiply the Celsius temperature by $\dfrac{9}{5}$.

3. Add 32 to that product.

Example 2:   Convert 17°C to Fahrenheit.

STEP 1. Substitute 17 for the letter C in the formula $F = \dfrac{9}{5}C + 32$.

$$F = \dfrac{9}{5}C + 32$$

$$F = \dfrac{9}{5}(17) + 32$$

STEP 2. Write 17 in fraction form.

$$F = \left(\dfrac{9}{5} \times \dfrac{17}{1}\right) + 32$$

STEP 3. Perform the operation in parenthesis first. Multiply the fractions.

$$F = \dfrac{153}{5} + 32$$

STEP 4. Change the improper fraction to a decimal number.

$$F = 30.6 + 32$$

STEP 5. Add 30.6 to the 32.

$$F = 62.6$$

The answer is 62.6°F.

Here is another method for performing temperature conversions. Let us see how these conversions work by using a conversion we know: normal body temperature (98.6°F equals 37°C).

If you are given °F, follow these steps:

1. Subtract 32.
2. Multiply by 5.
3. Divide by 9.

Example 3: Convert 98.6° Fahrenheit to Celsius

STEP 1. Subtract 32.

$$98.6 - 32 = 66.6$$

STEP 2. Multiply by 5.

$$66.6 \cdot 5 = 333$$

STEP 3. Divide by 9.

$$333 \div 9 = 37$$

The answer is 37°C.

The answer checks since 98.6°F = 37°C.

If you are given °C, follow these steps:

1. Multiply by 9.
2. Divide by 5.
3. Add 32.

Example 4: Convert 37° Celsius to Fahrenheit

STEP 1. Multiply by 9.

$$37 \cdot 9 = 333$$

STEP 2. Divide by 5.

$$333 \div 5 = 66.6$$

STEP 3. Add 32.

$$66.6 + 32 = 98.6$$

The answer is 98.6°F.

The answer checks since 37°C = 98.6°F.

Index

Note: Page numbers followed by "f" and "t" indicate figures and tables, respectively.